MUSCLE AND ITS DISEASES
An Outline Primer of Basic Science and Clinical Method

MUSCLE AND ITS DISEASES
An Outline Primer of Basic Science and Clinical Method

Irwin M. Siegel, M.D.
Associate Professor, Departments of Orthopaedic Surgery and Neurological Sciences, Rush-Presbyterian-St. Luke's Medical Center; Lecturer, Department of Orthopaedic Surgery, Abraham Lincoln School of Medicine, University of Illinois at Chicago; Senior Attending Orthopaedic Surgeon and Chairman, Department of Orthopaedic Surgery, Strauss Surgical Group Association, S.C., Louis A. Weiss Memorial Hospital; Director, Muscle Disease Clinics, University of Illinois Medical Center at Chicago and Louis A. Weiss Memorial Hospital; Co-Director, Muscle Disease Clinic, Rush-Presbyterian-St. Luke's Medical Center, Chicago, Illinois

YEAR BOOK MEDICAL PUBLISHERS, INC.
Chicago • London

Library of Congress Cataloging-in-Publication Data

Siegel, Irwin M., 1927–
  Muscle and its diseases.

  Includes bibliographies and index.
  1. Neuromuscular diseases—Outlines, syllabi, etc.
I. Title. [DNLM: 1. Muscular Diseases. WE 550 S571m]
RC925.S473 1986   616.7'4   86-13314
ISBN 0-8151-7653-8

Sponsoring Editor: Richard H. Lampert
Manager, Copyediting Services: Frances M. Perveiler
Copyeditor: Francis A. Byrne
Production Project Manager: Etta Worthington
Proofroom Supervisor: Shirley E. Taylor

1234567890YC90,89,88,87,86

For all the children—theirs, and mine as well

"The contemplation of things as they are, without error or confusion, without substitution or imposture, is in itself a nobler thing than a whole harvest of invention."

Francis Bacon (1561–1626)

"Whatever can be said at all can be said clearly, and whatever cannot be said clearly should not be said at all."

Ludwig Wittgenstein (1889–1951)

"The kind of life lived by a patient under conditions of vigorous response to a challenge is infinitely preferable to a crunching, desperate winding-down."

Norman Cousins (Human Options)

PREFACE

This monograph has been written in response to the needs of students and practitioners who require a complete yet concise outline of muscle and its diseases, without reviewing the prodigious body of literature now available on the subject. The format stresses the close relation between underlying pathogenic mechanisms and biomechanical correlates with clinical manifestations and treatment. It is written for those who:

- Want a problem-oriented bedside manual for ready reference;
- Wish to review the subject in brief;
- Want to correlate the clinical with the basic sciences;
- Find an outline of diagnosis and state-of-the-art treatment of practical value.

The book does not:

- Present a comprehensive review of the literature;
- Examine the vast body of current ongoing research;
- Discuss any single topic in depth;
- Outline processes or procedures beyond the detail necessary for an understanding of their practical application.

Though compendious, the text includes such materials as are necessary to understand, diagnose, and treat the majority of muscle diseases. Topics are presented where deemed pertinent, although when a subject is related to several headings its exposition may be shared. Overlap has not been avoided where necessary but some material has been duplicated for emphasis. The expanded outline form was chosen for readability and ease of reference. Part I (Basic Science) reviews the anatomy, chemistry, and physiology of muscle, setting the stage for a presentation of relevant techniques for clinical and laboratory diagnosis in Part II, classification in Part III, and a survey of management in Part IV. A Bibliography appears at the end of each part. Relevant illustrations are placed adjacent to related text when possible, much as in a slide lecture. Wherever feasible, clinical observations have been related to basic science processes.

IRWIN M. SIEGEL, M.D.

ACKNOWLEDGMENTS

I wish to thank the following people for their assistance in the preparation of this book:

- Ms. Jackie Hagedorn and Mrs. Alice Thanner, for expert secretarial service and proofing of the manuscript.
- Miss Iris Sachs, for bibliographic assistance.
- Muscular Dystrophy Association of America, for generous encouragement and support.
- Dr. Victor Dubowitz and Dr. Michael Brooke, for continuing tuition in the fascinating field of myology.
- Dr. Russell Glantz, for ongoing instruction in the intricacies of neurological diagnosis.
- The clinic staffs of the muscle disease clinics of the Rush-Presbyterian-St. Luke's Medical Center, The University of Illinois Abraham Lincoln School of Medicine, and The Louis A. Weiss Memorial Hospital for their able help with the multidisciplined management of the patient roster and for shared instruction in their separate disciplines.
- Orthotists Oscar and Michael Silverman, for editorial assistance in the area of their expertise.
- Artist Kurt Peterson, for his outstanding illustrations.
- Joseph Fortman, for assistance with photography.
- My wife, Barbara, for accepting with understanding the homebound weekends and evenings apart while I isolated myself to work and rework the manuscript.
- The Year Book Medical Publishers of Chicago and particularly Richard Lampert, Editor-in-Chief, Text and Reference Publishing, for patiently and skillfully shepherding the book through editing and publication.

IRWIN M. SIEGEL, M.D.

CONTENTS

Introduction

Muscle: (from the Greek), a mouse. Probably so named because of its quick movements and the similarity of tendon to tail.
• Accounts for 45% of body weight in man;
• Is the body's largest tissue;
• With the help of electrical (neural) input, converts chemical energy to mechanical work while it gives off heat (and does this silently);
• Can be switched on within milliseconds;
• Utilizes both carbohydrate and fats as fuel;
• Can operate aerobically (with oxygen) and anaerobically (without oxygen);
• Has a built-in servomechanism;
• Accomplishes its work at 40% efficiency (approximately that of a Diesel engine); and
• Is good to eat.*

Muscle diseases have increasingly engaged the attention and efforts of pediatricians, internists, orthopedic surgeons, psychiatrists, and physicians in related specialties. Children with muscle disease are often misdiagnosed early and may see at least several physicians before a correct diagnosis is made. This needlessly delays vital genetic counseling and sometimes important therapy.

Table 1 contains the prevalence and incidence of some common

*With thanks to D.R. Wilkie, who, in the 1960s, concluded an advertisement for a lecture on muscle with this laconic remark.

TABLE 1.
Muscular Disease: Prevalence and Incidence

MUSCULAR DISEASE	PREVALENCE†	INCIDENCE‡
Duchenne muscular dystrophy*	28–66	168–279
Limb-girdle dystrophy		
Autosomal recessive	12	38
Sporadic	8	27
Becker	18	28
Facioscapulohumeral	2–6	4–9
Dystrophia myotonica	24–55	135
Myotonica congenita	5	5

*Based on one million male cases at birth.
†Per million living cases.
‡Per million births.
The mutation rate in DMD is 89/million gametes; in Limb-Girdle Dystrophy 31/million gametes; in FSH 5/10 million gametes.

muscular diseases. Although the causes and cures of these diseases are not known, three major theories have been proposed to explain their pathogenesis: (1) abnormal vascularity; (2) abnormal neuronal influence; and (3) abnormal muscle metabolism. However, incurable is not synonymous with untreatable. This book was written to assist the practitioner in accurately reaching a diagnosis and applying treatment appropriately.

Abbreviations Used Throughout the Text

ACH	Acetylcholine
ADP	Adenosine diphosphate
AFO	Ankle-foot orthosis
ALS	Amyotrophic lateral sclerosis
ANA	Antinuclear antibody
AP	Action potential
ATP	Adenosine triphosphate
BFAO	Balanced forearm orthosis
CG	Center of gravity
CMT	Charcot-Marie-Tooth disease
CNS	Central nervous system
CP	Creatine phosphate
CPK	Creatine phosphokinase
CVP	Central venous pressure
DM	Dystrophia myotonica
DMD	Duchenne muscular dystrophy
EMG	Electromyogram
EOM	Extraocular muscles
ESR	Erythrocyte sedimentation rate
FSH	Facioscapulohumeral dystrophy
HMSN	Hereditary motor and sensory neuropathy
IPPB	Intermittent positive pressure breathing
KAFO	Knee-ankle-foot orthosis

LDH	Lactic dehydrogenase
LE	Lupus erythematosus
LGD	Limb girdle dystrophy
NCV	Nerve conduction velocity
SCM	Sternocleidomastoid
SGOT	Serum glutamic oxaloacetic transaminase
SGPT	Serum glutamic pyruvic transaminase
SMA	Spinal muscular atrophy
SR	Sarcoplasmic reticulum
TDL	Tasks of daily living
TLSO	Thoraco-lumbo-sacral orthosis
UCB	University of California Berkeley (orthosis)
VC	Vital capacity
WBC	White blood count

PART I

Basic Science

Functional Anatomy

"Anatomy is to physiology as geography to history: It describes the theatre of events."

Jean Fernel (1497–1558), *On the Natural Part of Medicine*

A contractile system requires (1) a molecular mechanism for contraction, (2) a method of stimulating and regulating that mechanism, (3) a source of energy, (4) a way of coupling that energy to the contractile elements, and (5) a method for joining those elements to the part to be moved.

There are approximately 450 skeletal muscles in the human body (Fig 1–1). These vary in size from the stapedius muscle (only a few millimeters long) to the gluteus maximus. They comprise 45% of the body's weight (23% in infants) and utilize 45% of the body's metabolism. The ratio of muscle to bone mass remains relatively constant (15 to 20) throughout the upper and lower limbs, even though the legs contain three times as much muscle and bone as the arms. Cross-sectional area is related inversely to fiber length and directly to muscle weight. The total physiological cross-section of all the muscles in the human body is about six square feet. The overall maximum tension a muscle can generate is equal to a force of approximately 45 lb/square inch. If the one-quarter billion skeletal muscle fibers of the body all contracted maximally at the same time, they would produce a force of 25 tons.

FIG 1–1.

(450) SKELETAL MUSCLES
45 { % body's weight % metabolism lb/in^2 force

I. The fundamental properties of muscle.
   A. Excitability—the ability to respond to a stimulus.
   B. Contractility—the ability to produce tension.
      1. A muscle's primary function is to generate force. Thus, movements of specific parts of the skeleton are produced or prevented.
      2. Muscles cross one or more joints and are attached to bone by tendons.
II. The structure and form of muscle.
   A. The cells of all skeletal muscles are similar in structure and contractile mechanism.
   B. Range, power and precision depend upon the three-dimensional fascicular arrangement of muscle fibers.
      1. Muscle fibers can shorten to approximately 60% of their resting length (the ideal length at which maximum tension can be developed). For example, peak tension for the quadriceps muscle is generated from 10 degrees of knee flexion. Thus, two factors control the degree to which a muscle can flex a joint.
         a) Length of the muscle.
         b) Distance of muscle insertion from the joint.
            (1) The length of muscle necessary to achieve full flexion increases as the point of its insertion on the distal bone moves away from the joint. A short muscle, to achieve full flexion by contracting 60% of its length, must insert close to the joint; a long muscle may insert further away. Where muscle fibers run the full length of muscle (as tends to be the case in fusiform [spindle-shaped] muscles such as biceps or triceps brachii), a muscle may insert 25% of its length away from the joint (Fig 1–2). If the length of the short lever arm on the distal bone exceeds a quarter of the length of the muscle, contraction will be inadequate to achieve full joint flexion or exten-

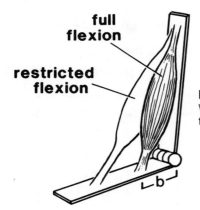

full flexion

restricted flexion

FIG 1–2.
When b is greater than 25% of muscle length, full flexion is not possible.

Lb

sion. Therefore, muscles tend to lie parallel to long bones because maximal efficiency of muscle size is gained when they insert close to the joint.

(2) Lever arm lengths acted on by muscle and overall length of muscle are fixed anatomical characteristics (Fig 1–3). In performance, this is an area where heredity may affect skill, some individuals having dimensions more effective than others for the accomplishment of certain tasks. However, most physical endeavors utilize multiple limb segments, and here skill predominates. The overall muscular moment applied to an activity can be varied by adjusting effective limb length through interactions at several joints as well as varying joint position to effect the angle of pull of muscles on joint segments. Thus, limb dynamics are adjusted for optimum performance.

(3) Some muscles seem best suited to produce acceleration along the arc of motion of the joint (spurt muscles such as the biceps brachii and brachialis) (Fig 1–4). Others lie parallel to the long axis of the moving bone and act to provide a stabilizing force during a rapid movement (shunt muscles, such as the brachioradialis).

III. The function and performance of muscle.

A. Parallel fibers are found in fusiform muscles (such as the biceps or triceps brachii). These muscles are capable of quick bursts of activity over the greatest range of contraction.

B. Fasciculi oblique to the line of pull can increase the number of muscle fibers without unduly increasing the muscle's diameter.
   1. Penniform (feather-shaped: unipennate, bipennate, multipennate), such as deltoid, provide multiple short fibers that

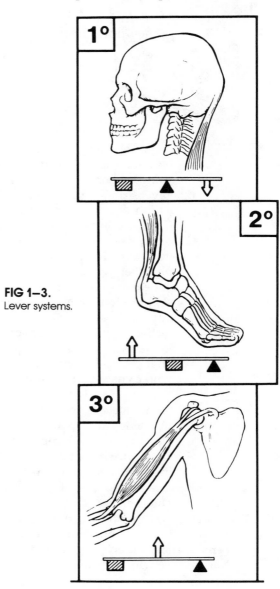

FIG 1–3.
Lever systems.

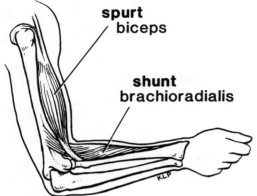

spurt
biceps

shunt
brachioradialis

FIG 1–4.
Accelerating and stabilizing
muscles.

can generate more tension per unit of whole muscle (Fig
1–5). In such muscles, fibers are attached to a septa in a
feather-like manner at an angle to the line of action. These
muscles are slow but capable of powerful contraction because more fibers participate in a maximum contraction
that can be maintained by some fibers while others are at
rest.

2. Muscular tension is a function of the number of sarcomeres
   in parallel. Shortening velocity is related to the number of
   sarcomeres in series. The larger the angle of pinnation (to
   tendon of insertion), the less are the tension and shortening velocity of the muscle fiber.
3. Similar fiber lengths are seen within muscles performing a
   synergistic function (e.g., ankle dorsiflexors have fibers

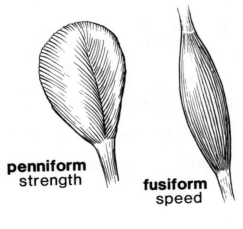

penniform
strength

fusiform
speed

FIG 1–5.
Fascicular form and function.

endomysium

perimysium

epimysium

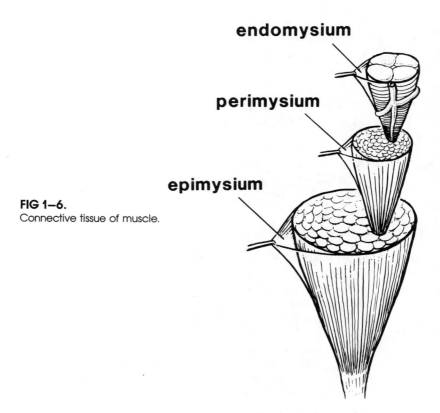

FIG 1–6.
Connective tissue of muscle.

twice the length of plantar flexors). These architectural considerations are important when planning tendon transfers to substitute for or supplant the motor activity of a given muscle.

4. By and large, the number of muscle fibers does not increase after the neonatal period. Increase in muscular size is due to enlargement of fibers.

IV. Connective tissue of muscles.
  A. Components.
    1. Epimysium—continuous layer of deep fascia surrounding the anatomical muscle.
    2. Perimysium—macroscopically subdivides muscle into fiber bundles (fasciculi).
    3. Endomysium—surrounds individual muscle fibers (muscle cellular units) binding them together and to perimysium (Fig 1–6).

B. Functions.
1. Constitute pathways for nerves and blood vessels.
2. Determine the extent of stretching and deformability in a muscle because connective tissue is more resistant to stretching than other constituents of muscle.
3. Constitute the "series elastic element"* (as contrasted with the "parallel elastic element" [capillaries, tracheoles, sarcoplasmic reticulum, sarcolemma], also a noncontractile compartment), which, acting as a spring, transmits the forces generated by muscle.
4. Provide tendon to anchor muscle to bone at origin and insertion.

BIBLIOGRAPHY

Clemente CD (ed): *Gray's Anatomy*, ed 13. Philadelphia, Lea & Febiger, 1985, pp 429–436.
Cochran G: *A Primer of Orthopaedic Biomechanics*. New York, Churchill Livingstone, Inc, 1982.
Cruess RL: *The Musculoskeletal System: Embryology, Biochemistry, and Physiology*. New York, Churchill Livingstone, Inc, 1982.
Donohoe KM: *An overview of neuromuscular disease*. Nurs Clin North Am 1979; 14:95–106.
Owen R, Goodfellow J, Bullough P: *Scientific Foundations of Orthopaedics and Traumatology*. Philadelphia, WB Saunders Co, 1980.
Rosse C, Clawson D: *The Musculoskeletal System in Health and Disease*. New York, Harper & Row, 1980.
Wickiewicz T, et al: *Muscle Architecture of the Human Lower Limb. Corr* 1983; 179:275–283.
Wilson F: *The Musculoskeletal System: Basic Processes and Disorders*. Philadelphia, JB Lippincott, Co, 1982.

*The "series elastic element" also has a major component in the cross-bridges.

2

Histology

"An organ is a cell state in which every cell is a citizen."
Rudolph Virchow (1821–1902)

A single skeletal muscle cell is called a muscle fiber. This fiber is the unit of structure in physiologic response. The number of fibers in a muscle depends mostly on its size (biceps—2,600,000; stapedius—1,500). Fibers are grouped into bundles (fascicles). Some muscles have small fascicles (fine grain), such as the ocular muscles; others (e.g., gluteal muscles) have large fascicles and show a coarse grain. Although some fibers may extend the entire length of a fascicle and attach at each end (it is commonly held that most fascicles longer than 5 cm contain no fibers extending their entire length), others attach at one end only or lie wholly within the fascicle, without attachment at either end.

A muscle fiber is:

I. 10–100 microns in diameter.
   A. Thickness varies with type of muscle and even within the same muscle. For example, ocular muscles have fine fibers, whereas the deltoid has coarse fibers. Fiber diameter increases with age, exercise, and the influence of male sexual hormones. An adult fiber may grow to 10 times its diameter at birth. Exercise can increase fiber size by 25%.

II. A multinucleated (about 35 per mm) long cell
   A. Longer fibers occur in nontapering muscles (e.g., sartorius).
III. An assembly of contractile protein surrounded by sarcolemma, an electrically polarized membrane that has the capacity to propagate an action potential.
IV. Composed of 75% water, 20% protein (80% fibrillar contractile protein, 20% water-soluble protein), and 1% glycogen.
V. A system composed of subunits called myofibrils. Myofibrils are 1–3 μ long, longitudinally arranged cylinders. These are:
   A. Surrounded by sarcoplasmic reticulum, a system of specialized smooth membrane-lined tubules (endoplasmic reticulum) periodically distributed lengthwise throughout the myofibril (Fig 2–1). At each end of a set of the sarcoplasmic reticulum, there is an enlargement called the terminal cisternae. The combination of the terminal cisternae and the transverse tubules that penetrate a muscle fiber form a triad.
   B. Composed of two types of longitudinally disposed contractile protein filamentous subunits in overlapping array, the thick (1.5 μ × 100 A) and thin (1.0 μ × 50 A) myofilaments. Cross-banding of these filaments in register in adjacent myofibrils gives a cross-striated appearance to the entire muscle fiber as revealed by the electron microscope. Mitochondria are located between myofibrils.
      1. The thick filaments are myosin.
      2. The thin filaments are chiefly actin, associated with tropomyosin and troponin.
      3. Interdigitation of the thick and thin filaments produces:
         a) Light bands (I-bands)—isotropic to polarized light—thin filament alone.
         b) Dark bands (A-bands)—anisotropic to polarized light—thick and thin filaments in overlap.
            (1) The actin filaments are attached to each other at the Z-line (Fig 2–2). The distance from one Z-line to the next (2.5 μ) constitutes a single sarcomere, the unit of structure and function within the myofibril. Each muscle fiber contains approximately 20,000 sarcomeres. In fast moving muscles (e.g., intrinsic hand musculature), sarcomeres are shorter (more contractile units per mm). When a muscle fiber is stretched, the ends of the actin filaments pull apart, leaving a light area in the center of the A-band. This is called

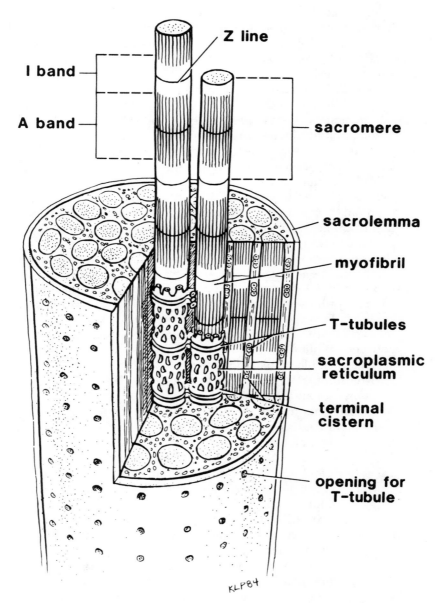

FIG 2–1.
Myofibrils and sarcoplasmic reticulum.

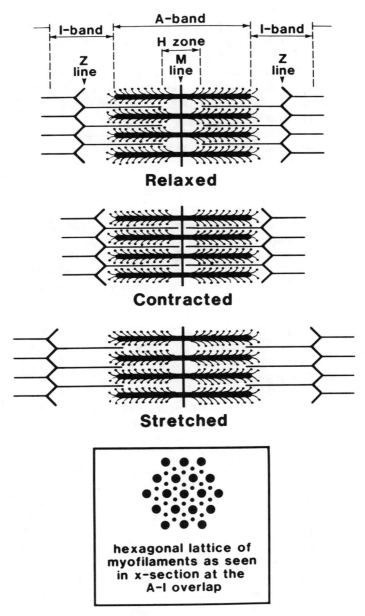

FIG 2–2.
Banding characteristics of muscle.

the H-zone. The M-line (400–800 A) is a dense line in the mid H-zone.

4. Summary of band characteristics (resting muscle).
    a) A—1.5 μ, anisotropic dark bands. Thick and thin filaments overlap.
    b) I—0.375 μ, isotropic light bands, thin filaments.
    c) Z—500–800 A—attachment for thin filaments.
    d) H—0.35 μ light zone in the middle of the A-band
    e) M—400–800 A, dense line in the mid H-zone.
5. Contractile proteins.
    a) Myosin—54%, in thick myofilaments with polarity (direction of force produced) reversed on each side of an M-band. Cross bridges with ATPase activity and a binding site for actin are present.
    b) Actin—25%. Thin filaments. Activates myosin ATPase.
    c) Tropomyosin—5%–11%. Found in thin filaments.
    d) Troponin—found in thin filaments.
        (1) Troponin and tropomyosin act to block actin binding to myosin. Together they comprise the relaxing protein system.
    e) Alpha actinin. Z-line.
    f) Beta actinin. Free end of actin.
    g) M-line protein. Cross bridges in the M-line connecting thick myofilaments.
    h) Component protein. Thick filaments.
6. Molecular structure of myofilaments.
    a) The myosin molecule has two globular heads that are directed toward the actin filaments (Fig 2–3). Myosin molecules aggregate in a reverse polarity on each side of the sarcomere (Fig 2–4).
    b) The actin molecules intertwine helically to constitute the actin filament (two strands of F [fibrous] actin, composed of many G [globular] actin subunits per filament). Bound to the surface of the actin filament are two proteins (Fig 2–5):
        (1) Tropomyosin—extends length of thin filament.
        (2) Troponin—present once per turn of helix.
    c) Six actin filaments surround a centrally placed myosin filament in a hexagonal lattice.
C. During shortening, actin and myosin filaments slide past one another, making and breaking contact (ratchet-gearing effect) between the myosin cross bridges and myosin binding sites

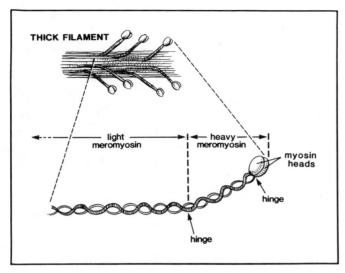

FIG 2–3.
Myosin molecule.

on the actin molecules of the six surrounding thin filaments, causing a change in length of the I- and H-bands.

MOTOR END PLATE

This mediates motor activity by generating an action potential at the neuromuscular junction, which is then propagated into the muscle fiber along the transverse tubular system (Fig 2–6). A terminal nerve twig loses its myelin sheath (and neurolemma in part) and forms a plaque about midway along a muscle fiber. The bulbous axonal-twig, which contains mitochondria and vesicles (containing acetylcholine, the chemical mediator that induces contraction, released on arrival of the nerve impulse), terminates directly on the sarcolemma. At the junc-

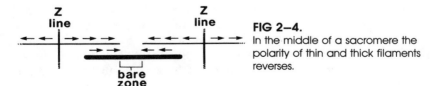

FIG 2–4.
In the middle of a sacromere the polarity of thin and thick filaments reverses.

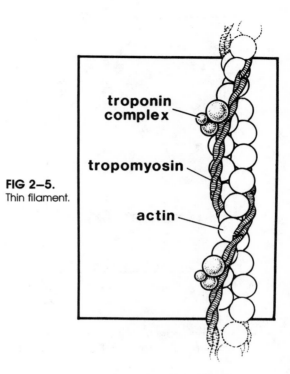

FIG 2–5.
Thin filament.

troponin complex

tropomyosin

actin

tional area, the sarcolemma is folded into troughs that contain acetylcholine receptor sites. Usually, a single branching nerve fiber innervates many (up to several hundred) muscle fibers. In muscles with precise movements, individual nerve fibers branch less. Healthy neurons exert a trophic influence which, through electrochemical nourishment, maintains muscle fibers in good condition.

MUSCLE SPINDLES

These are fusiform structures (Fig 2–7) interspersed in parallel orientation among skeletal muscle fibers, their several poles anchored to endo- and perimysium. Passive stretch places spindles under tension; muscle contraction relieves tension. A spindle consists of 2 to 12 specialized muscle fibers (intrafusal fibers) enclosed in a connective tissue capsule. Spindles are surrounded by skeletomotor (extrafusal) fibers. Both sensory and motor nerves penetrate the spindle to terminate on the intrafusal fibers. The intrafusal fibers are striated muscle, but their

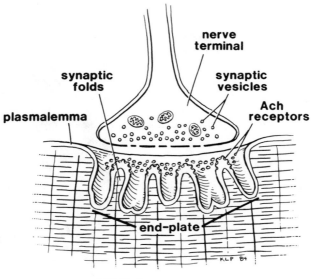

FIG 2–6.
Neuromuscular junction.

equatorial zone is largely devoid of striations and dilated by the accumulation of nuclei.

In some fibers, nuclei occupy a central sarcoplasmic bag (nuclear bag fibers), in others a core chain (nuclear chain fiber). The nuclear bag is most sensitive to rapid stretch. Each spindle has a large afferent nerve fiber that wraps around the nuclear bags (and central nuclear chain fibers) as the primary annulospiral endings. Secondary afferent nerve fibers terminate on the polar segments of nuclear chain fibers. Afferent nerve fibers are sensitive to changes in both velocity and amplitude of muscle stretch.

Intrafusal fiber contraction is initiated by fusimotor fibers (gamma efferents) that enter the spindle and terminate by motor end plates on the polar segments of the intrafusal spindle fibers. Spindles are the muscle's length-registering receptors. The activity of the muscle spindle stretch receptor and gamma efferent system subserve those reflexes (such as stretch reflexes) underlying the fine control of movement. Although many muscle spindles are found in the intrinsic muscles of the hand, there are more per unit muscle tissue in the neck than anywhere else in the body. This is because neck musculature plays such an important role in maintaining posture. Pathological changes in muscle spindles can occur in various disease states.

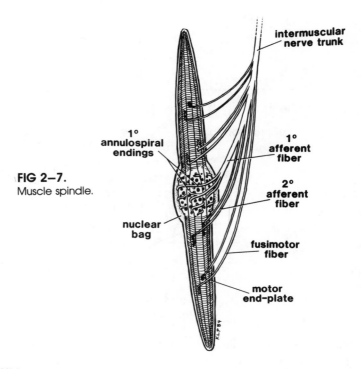

intermuscular
nerve trunk

1°
annulospiral
endings

1°
afferent
fiber

2°
afferent
fiber

FIG 2–7.
Muscle spindle.

nuclear
bag

fusimotor
fiber

motor
end-plate

BIBLIOGRAPHY

Arey LB: *Human Histology.* Philadelphia, WB Saunders Co, 1974.

Flickinger C, Brown J, Kutchai H, et al: *Medical Cell Biology.* Philadelphia, WB Saunders Co, 1979.

Ham A, Cormack D: *Histology,* ed 8. Philadelphia, JB Lippincott, Co, 1979.

Hopkins C: *Structure and Function of Cells.* Philadelphia, WB Saunders Co, 1978.

Kakulas BA, Adams RD: *Disease of Muscle,* ed 4. New York, Harper & Row, 1985, pp 85–98.

Stryer L: *Biochemistry.* San Francisco, WH Freeman & Co, 1981.

3

Development, Growth, and Regeneration of Muscle

"Nature is sufficient in all for all."

Hippocrates (460?–377? B.C.),
Nutriment, XV (Translation by W. H. S. Jones)

Skeletal muscle is derived from mesenchyma (myotomes).

I. Presumptive myoblasts differentiate into myoblasts that fuse into myotubes, each of which develops into a muscle fiber (Fig 3–1).
   A. The total number of muscle fibers is established at birth.
   B. Growth is achieved by addition of new sarcomeres (axial) or increase in the number of myofibrils (girth), and is stimulated by:
      1. Neurotropic influences. Initially the peripheral nervous system and skeletal muscles develop independently. However, unless muscle becomes innervated, its rate of growth is greatly retarded.
      2. Stretch.
      3. Hormonal factors.

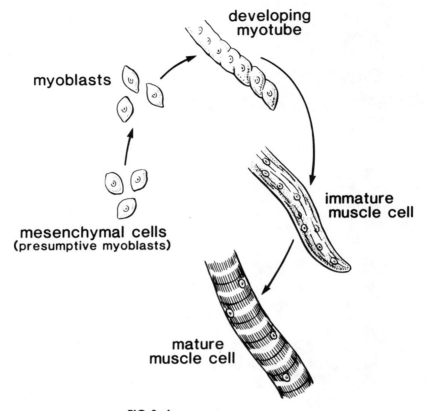

FIG 3–1.
Skeletal muscle fiber development.

C. Abnormal myogenesis is thought to cause morphologically specific myopathies (Table 3–1).

D. Approximately 50% of the body's skeletal muscle undergoes "turnover" in one to two weeks. (Amino acids $\overset{Ks}{\underset{Kd}{\rightleftharpoons}}$ protein, where Ks = synthesis and Kd = degeneration; Kto = Ks/Kd, where Kto = turnover. In muscular dystrophy, Kd exceeds Ks.)

II. Regeneration.

A. Satellite cells are reserved cells that retain stem cell potential for generating muscle cells (Fig 3–2).

TABLE 3–1.
Morphologically Specific Defects Occurring During Embryonic Muscle Development

DEVELOPMENTAL STAGE	DEVELOPMENTAL ACTIVITY	LOCALIZATION OF DEVELOPMENTAL DEFECT
Premyoblastic (0–1 mo.)	Mesenchymal cells	
Myoblastic (1–2 mo.)	Multiplication and fusion; contractile protein synthesis	
Myotubular (2–4 mo.)	Sarcomere formation and growth; central nuclei-fascicular differentiation	Myotubular myopathy; Centronuclear myopathies
Immature myocytic (4–5 mo.)	Nuclear margination; organelle dispersion	
Early and late histochemical (5–7 mo.)	Neural control; fiber type differentiation; mosaic distribution	Type II predominance; structural changes (cores, rods, inclusion bodies)
Maturing myocytic (over 7+ mo.)	Morphological growth; histochemical maturation	Type I or Type II hypotrophy; structural changes

1. Failure of this process occurs in Duchenne muscular dystrophy and other neuromuscular diseases (Fig 3–3).
2. Subclinical denervation with secondary reinnervative grouping is a natural concomitant of aging in normal muscle. Lumbosacral motor unit dropout can cause up to 85% atrophy of the lower leg muscles after age 65.

THE MUSCLE TWITCH

There are fast and slow-twitch muscles in the body. Examples include:

I. Extraocular muscles—fast.
II. Postural muscles of the legs (e.g., soleus)—slow (Fig 3–4). "Fast" and "slow" muscles are determined on the basis of the nature of the fiber predominating in any given muscle. The motor nerve serving the fiber determines the type of a given fiber. In other words, a motor nerve innervates only one fiber type (Fig 3–5).
III. Changes in motor nerve supply can change fiber type characteristics of muscle cells.
IV. To a certain extent, changes in function (exercise) can alter fiber

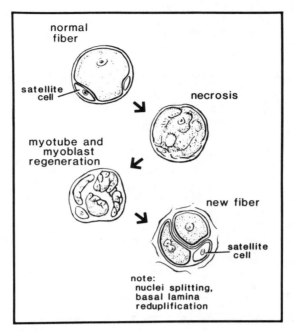

FIG 3–2.
Satellite cell function—fiber splitting.

type characteristics (see "Muscle Fiber Type and Activity" in section on Energy Metabolism).

V. In man, there are no muscles with pure fiber typing. However, certain muscles such as ankle dorsiflexors (tibialis anticus) that show moderately fast twitch, marked postactivation potentiation, and fatigue sensitivity, are 64% Type I fiber. In contrast, ankle plantar flexors (gastrocsoleus) are slow twitch, poor postactivation potential, fatigue resistant, and contain 76% Type I fiber.

VI. Characteristics of muscle fiber types* (Table 3–2).

A. Type I.

1. Smaller diameter, red, dark.

2. Slower contraction (twitch 100–120 msec). Sustained activity.

3. Derives energy predominantly from respiration (oxidative phosphorylation = aerobic, Krebs cycle).

   a) High content of oxidative enzymes.

---

*Fiber types differ principally in their biochemical machinery for handling energy substrates.

4. Mainly uses fatty acids and glucose for energy.
5. Rich in myoglobin and mitochondria.
6. Light-stained for myofibrillar ATPase activity (Ph 9.4).
B. Type II.
1. Larger diameter, white, pale (less capillary density).
2. Fewer mitochondria.
3. Fast contraction (40 msec), but short duration of activity.

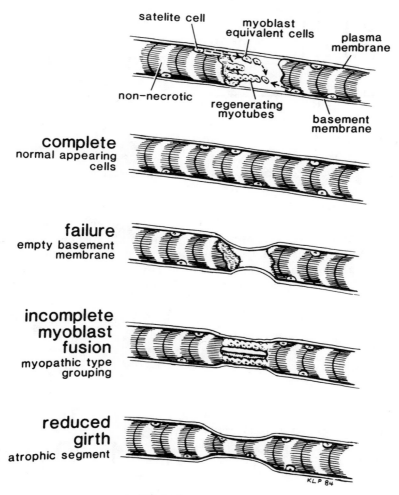

FIG 3–3.
Muscle fiber regeneration.

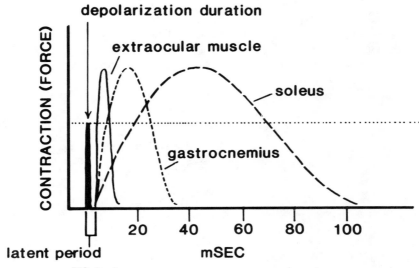

FIG 3—4.
Isometric contraction duration in various types of muscle.

4. Metabolic characteristic: Glycolysis (anaerobic) and lactase production more prominent. Uses glycogen for energy.
5. Myofibrillar ATPase activity higher on histochemical staining. Stains dark (pH 9.4).
6. Sarcoplasmic reticulum allows activation of actin-myosin filaments at a faster rate. Thus, more tension can be developed at faster velocities.
7. Type II fibers can be subdivided into Types IIA, IIB, and

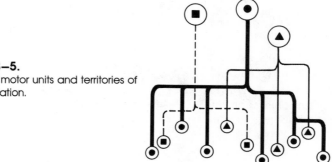

FIG 3—5.
Three motor units and territories of innervation.

TABLE 3–2.
Characteristics of Skeletal Muscle Fibers

CATEGORY	TYPE I	TYPE II
Size	I < II (cross section)	II > I
Color (macroscopic)	Red	White
Contractile properties	Slow but sustained activity	Fast but short duration activity
Metabolic characteristics	Oxidative phosphorylation (Aerobic-Krebs cycle) uses fatty acids and glucose	Glycolysis (anaerobic) uses glycogen, pyruvate lactate
Mitochondrial enzymes		
NADH	+ + +	+
Cytochrome oxidase	+ + +	+
SDH	+ + +	+
LDH	+	+ + +
GPM	+	+ + +
Phosphorylase (glycolytic enzyme)	+	+ + +
Myofibrillary ATPase (pH 9.5)	+	+ + +
Glycogen (PAS)	+	+ + +
FAT (Oil Red O)	+ + +	+
Myoglobin	High	Low
Specific example	Soleus	Biceps brachii

IIC on the basis of oxidative enzyme content and can be trained for some oxidative capacity.

BIBLIOGRAPHY

Adams RD: Principles of myopathology and principles of clinical mycology: Thayer lectures. *Hopkins Med J* 1972; 131:24–62.

Dhoot GK: Initiation of differentiation into skeletal muscle fiber types. *Muscle Nerve* 1985; 8:307–316.

Pette D, Vrbova G: Neural control of phenotype expression in mammalian muscle fibers. *Muscle Nerve* 1985; 8:676–689.

Poland J, Hobart D, Payton O: *The Musculoskeletal System*, ed 2. New York, Medical Examination Publishing Co, 1981.

Schmidt H, Emser W: Regeneration of frog twitch and slow muscle fibers after mincing. *Muscle Nerve* 1985; 8:633–643.

Walton JN (ed): *Disorders of Voluntary Muscles*, ed. 4. New York, Churchill Livingstone, Inc, 1981.

4

Molecular Basis of Muscle Contraction

"Love may make the world go round, but muscle gives it the push."
M. Brooke

I. During muscle contraction, sliding of the two filaments occurs because of the cyclic interaction (make and break contraction) between proteins on the thick (myosin cross bridges) and thin (actin) filaments.

   A. Sarcoplasmic reticulum surrounds myofibrils with a canalicular network (Table 4–1). This consists of longitudinal tubules adjacent to the A-bands and terminal cisternae at the Z-band or AI junctions. Two terminal cisternae or lateral tubules and a T-tubule (the T-system connects to the cell membrane) comprise a triad. A depolarizing wave begins at the motor end plate and spreads over the muscle cell membrane and into the T-system (Fig 4–1). This wave of depolarization causes a release of calcium from the terminal cisternae into the triads (Fig 4–2). Action potentials and membrane potentials in muscle surface

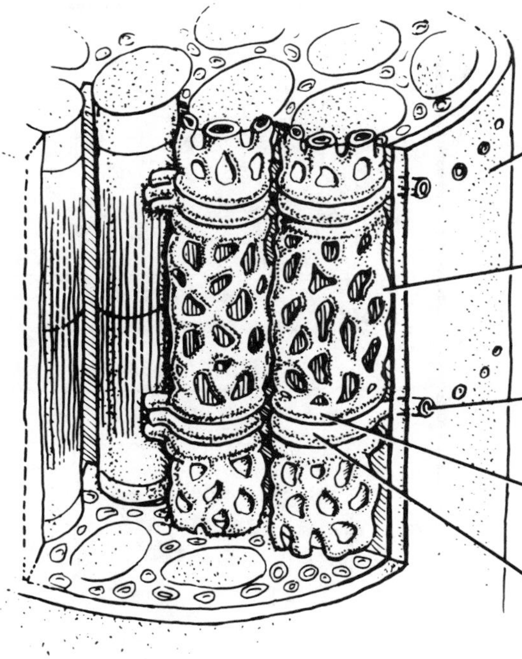
sacrolemma
sacroplastic reticulum
opening to T–tubule
terminal cistern
T–tubule

FIG 4–1.
T-tubule system.

membrane are produced by a process analogous to that seen in nerve. In each case, the membrane potential results from the combined effect of concentration gradients of sodium and potassium across the membrane and the relative membrane permeability to each of these ions.

B. Troponin and tropomyosin mediate calcium ion regulation of muscle contraction as tropomyosin sterically blocks actin. Troponin is unique in having three sites of interaction; one with calcium molecules, a second with tropomyosin, and a third with actin (Fig 4–3). Thus, calcium ion inactivates the inhibitory action of the tropomyosin-troponin system* and also activates the energy-transducing enzyme myosin ATPase. Actin and myosin join, the myosin heads now interacting with actin units of the thin filaments (Fig 4–4). When calcium levels are below

*In binding to troponin, calcium shifts tropomyosin, exposing the actin binding sites for myosin.

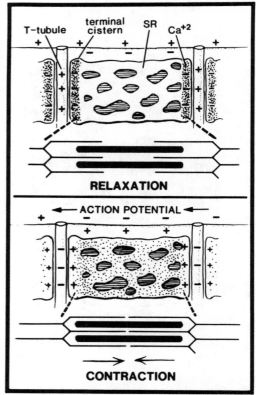

FIG 4—2.
Depolarization.

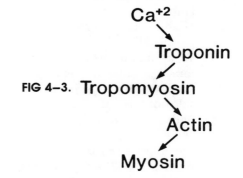

FIG 4–3.

TABLE 4–1.*
Functions of Muscle Membrane System

Sarcolemma
  Diffusion boundary
  Passive selective permeability
  Active ion transport
  Generation and propagation of the action potential (AP)
Sarcoplasmic Reticulum
  Active accumulation and sequestration of Ca^{2+}
  Rapid release of Ca^{2+} in response to activating signal
T-Tubular System
    Active conduction of surface AP into cell interior
    Link between sarcolemma and SR

*From Barchi RL, AAN Special Courses. Muscle Membranes and Muscle Diseases.

$10^{-7}M$, the interaction of actin and myosin is blocked: calcium levels above $10^{-5}M$ produce a maximum interaction between these molecules and allow peak tension to develop. Muscle tension is graded in this manner.
  C. Actin-myosin is a complex formed by strong bonds established

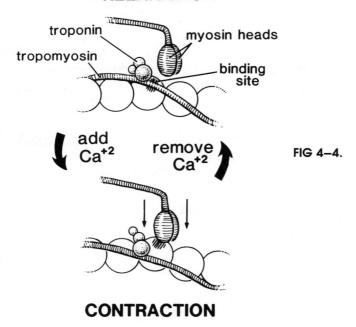

RELAXATION

troponin

tropomyosin

myosin heads

binding site

add Ca^{+2} remove Ca^{+2} FIG 4–4.

CONTRACTION

between binding sites on the myosin heads and binding sites on the actin molecules.

1. ATP dissociates this complex into actin and myosin (the ATP remains bound to the myosin).

a) The myosin ATP is hydrolyzed to produce ADP and inorganic phosphate.

b) The energy liberated by ATP provides a relative force between the two sets of filaments. The filaments have a polarity such that the thin filaments are propelled or slide toward the center of the thick filaments. The power strokes come from the tilting of the myosin head complex relative to actin (Fig 4–5). At constant length, such interactions occur a number of times at one site (isometric contraction). If the muscle shortens (isotonic contraction), such interactions take place consecutively at different

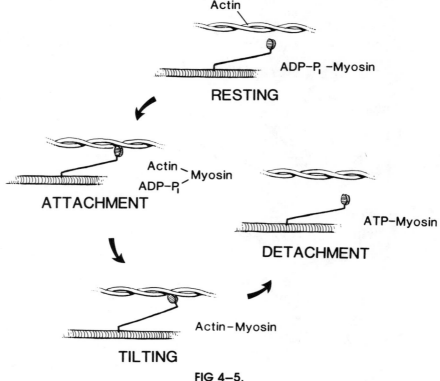

FIG 4–5.

sites. Thus, new cross bridge formation occurs along the thick filament.

c) Stated concisely, excitation contraction coupling is achieved by the control of sarcoplasmic calcium concentration. As calcium dissociates from troponin, the actin-myosin binding sites become covered once more by tropomyosin. After calcium is released, it is taken up again by the longitudinal tubules of the sarcoplasmic reticulum and the muscle relaxes. This is a process of active ionic transport against a concentration gradient.

BIBLIOGRAPHY

Davies RE: A molecular theory of muscle contraction. *Nature* 1963; 199:1068–1074.

Huxley HE: The contraction of muscle. *Scientific American* 1958; 199:67–82.

Korn ED: Biochemistry of actomyosin-dependent cell motility (a review). Proc Natl Acad Sci USA 1978; 75:588–599.

Lehninger A: *Biochemistry,* ed 2. New York, Worth Publications, Inc, 1975.

Obinata T, Maruyama K, Sugita H, et al: Dynamic aspects of structural proteins in vertebrate skeletal muscle. *Muscle Nerve* 1981; 4:456–488.

Porter KE, Franzini-Armstrong C: The sarcoplasmic reticulum. *Scientific American* 1965; 212:73–80.

Salmons S: The response of skeletal muscle to different patterns of use—some new developments and concepts in *Plasticity of Muscle.* New York, Walter de Gruyter, Inc, 1980, pp 387–399.

Seymour J, O'Brien EJ: The position of tropomyosin in muscle thin filaments. *Nature* 1980; 283:680–682.

West JB (ed): *Physiological Basis of Medical Practice (Best and Taylor),* ed 11. Baltimore, William and Wilkins, 1985, pp 58–106.

5

Energy Metabolism of Muscle

"The cell never acts. It reacts."

Ernest Haeckel (1834–1919)

Fatigue susceptibility in muscle varies. It relates to the capacity of muscle to use different energy sources. This ability is developed differently in Type I and Type II fibers. Further, the intensity and duration of exercise greatly influence the fiber types involved. Slow twitch fibers (Type I) are primarily used in submaximal endurance exercise; Type II fibers are selectively used for exercises performed at intensities above the aerobic threshold. This has been related to the order of recruitment of motor units by the CNS; the slow Type I fibers are first selected for low intensity exercise. As intensity increases, more Type II fibers are recruited.

ENERGY SOURCES*

I. ATP (adenosine triphosphate)—universal and immediate source for contraction and active movements of cations (Fig 5–1).

*Nuclear magnetic resonance is a new laboratory and clinical technique for understanding muscle energy metabolism and chemistry (see bibliography).

Phosphocreatine + ADP $\rightleftharpoons$ Creatine + ATP

$ATP + H_2O \longrightarrow ADP + H_3PO_4 + 12,000$ calories

Glucose + 2 ATP (or glycogen + 1 ATP)
$\xrightarrow{\text{anaerobic}}$ 2 Lactic Acid + 4 ATP

Glucose + 2 ATP (or glycogen + 1 ATP)
$\xrightarrow{\text{oxygen}}$ 6 CO_2 + 6 H_2O + 40 ATP

FFA $\xrightarrow{\text{oxygen}}$ CO_2 + H_2O + ATP

FIG 5–1.
Energy sources for muscle contraction. (From Ganong WF: *Review of Medical Physiology,* ed 11. Los Altos, California, Lange Medical Publications, 1983. Used by permission.)

A. All other forms of stored energy must be converted to ATP before use.
B. On energy release, ATP is hydrolyzed to ADP (adenosine diphosphate) and P (inorganic phosphate) (Figs 5–2 and 5–3).
C. ATP dissociates cross bridges between myosin and actin filaments. Lack of ATP prohibits breaking of these cross bridges, causing rigor (rigor mortis at death).
D. Chemical sources for replenishing ATP.
　　1. Creatine phosphate (phosphagen system).
　　　　a) Readily available (stored in muscle in only small amounts) and rapidly mobilized high energy phosphate compound supplying energy for vigorous, explosive type of activity lasting less than 30 seconds.
　　　　b) CPK (creatine phosphokinase) catalyzes transfer of high energy phosphate to ADP, thus rapidly resynthesizing ATP.
　　2. Anaerobic glycolysis.

$$ATP + H_2O \rightleftharpoons ADP + P_i + H^+$$ **FIG 5–2.**

FIG 5–3.

$$2ADP \rightleftharpoons ATP + AMP$$

    a) Primary energy source for vigorous activity from 30 to 90 seconds. Produces energy much faster than the aerobic process.

    b) Anaerobic metabolism of glycogen first to glucose (enzymes and substrate necessary for anaerobic breakdown of glycogen are located in sarcoplasm) and then to pyruvate and lactic acid.

    c) Accumulation of lactic acid leads to an oxygen debt and fatigue.

    d) The energy liberated per glucose molecule for ATP resynthesis is many times smaller than in the oxidative process.

        (1) Four moles ATP for each mole glucose degradated. Two moles ATP are spent in the process. Thus, a *net gain* of two moles ATP.

  3. Oxidative phosphorylation.

    a) For vigorous activity lasting more than 90 seconds.

    b) Confined to mitochondria.

    c) Uses carbohydrate, fat and protein for fuel.

        (1) Fatty acids used first. Glucose spared for CNS.

    d) Metabolites aerobically broken down in citric acid cycle and electron transport system. Glucose converted to pyruvate, and lactic acid not formed.

    e) A large amount of ATP is produced for each glucose molecule degraded (on average, 36 moles ATP for every mole glucose degraded).

    f) End products CO_2 and H_2O—excess energy released as heat (Table 5–1).

At rest, only the aerobic pathway is in operation and fatty acids are the preferred metabolic fuel. With exercise, the several anaerobic pathways come into play. In the first 5–10 minutes of moderate exercise, muscle glycogen is depleted. From 10–40 minutes, blood glucose is the major source of energy (its uptake increases 7–20 times). From 40 minutes to four hours, blood glucose (which peaks at 180 minutes) is used more than free fatty acids. After four hours of moderate exercise, the ratio reverses and free fatty acids are used more than blood glucose. Thus, one sees a shift from carbohydrate to lipid utilization in

TABLE 5–1.
Characteristics of the Three Energy Systems*

VARIABLE	PHOSPHAGEN SYSTEM (ATP + CP)	ANAEROBIC METABOLISM (GLYCOLYSIS)	AEROBIC METABOLISM (OXIDATIVE PHOSPHORYLATION)
Performance time	Immediate: Less than 30 sec	Rapid action: 30 sec–3 min	Slow Greater than 90 sec
Fuel	ATP + creatine phosphate	Glycogen	Carbohydrate, fat, and protein
Byproducts	ADP + C + P	Lactic acid	$CO_2 + H_2O$
Function	Short duration sprint activities, high-power output	Intermediate activities	Long-duration endurance activities, low-power output

*From Schutt RC, Fleck SJ: Production and utilization of energy in athletes. Orthop Clin North Am 1983; 14:459–467. Used by permission.

moderate exercise. Oxygen supply is an important factor for sustained muscular activity.

During exercise, both the aerobic and anaerobic processes (Fig 5–4) work in concert.* Creatine phosphate and anaerobic glycolysis provide initial energy while the body adjusts to bring more oxygen to the muscles requiring it. After use, creatine phosphate is resynthesized. ATP is used to convert creatine to creatine phosphate. Pyruvic acid can be processed in the aerobic pathway if enough oxygen is available. Otherwise, it is metabolized to lactic acid. With full operation (adequate oxygen) of the aerobic pathway, lactic acid can be transformed back to pyruvic acid (in the liver) which can then be utilized by the mitochondria to generate still more energy. The liver also manufactures glycogen from lactic acid, thus keeping its accumulation, with an increase of cellular acidity which interferes with glycolysis, under control. Muscle myoglobin (an oxygen carrier similar to hemoglobin) releases oxygen as required by the muscle cell, even when little oxygen is available from the blood. The net result of these operations is the creation of an aerobic steady state where lactic acid is disposed, creatine phosphate stores replenished, and the "oxygen debt" repaid.

*Although anaerobic metabolism generates less ATP for energy (7% of that netted from aerobic metabolism), it produces it faster. In the time it takes to aerobically degrade one mole of glucose to yield 36 moles of ATP, 32 moles of glucose can be anaerobically metabolized yielding (at two ATP each) a total of 64 moles of ATP.

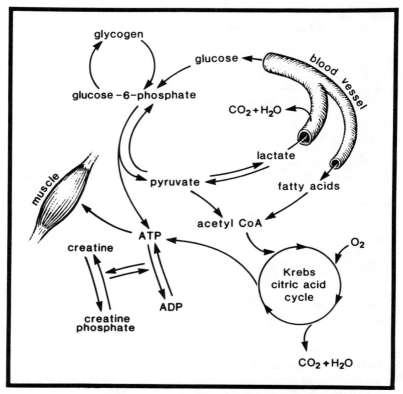

FIG 5–4.
Anaerobic and aerobic pathways.

This usually is achieved at exercise levels taxing no greater than 50% of an individual's maximal aerobic capacity. The contribution of energy systems to various athletic activities is listed in Table 5–2.

MUSCLE FIBER TYPE AND ACTIVITY

I. A motor nerve innervates only one fiber type. Slow twitch (Type I) motor units have smaller cell bodies; since they are more easily activated, not much input is required for a slow twitch muscle fiber to fire. In mild activity, slow twitch fibers are used. Since most of our everyday activities do not require major force, slow twitch fibers are better suited for continuous low-energy performance. To perform a simple task, such as drinking a glass of liquid, only about one-fifth of the maximal contraction capability of the arm is

TABLE 5–2.
Contribution (%) of Energy Systems in Various Athletics*

ACTIVITY	PHOSPHAGENS (ATP + CP)	ANAEROBIC METABOLISM (GLYCOLYTIC)	AEROBIC METABOLISM (OXIDATIVE)
Marathon	0	5	95
Running (1,500 m)	20	60	20
Swimming (440 yd)	20	40	40
Rowing	25	35	40
Cycling (road)	5	5	90
Recreational skiing	35	30	35
Baseball	80	20	0
Tennis	70	20	10
Golf	95	5	0
Volleyball	90	10	0
Weightlifting	98	2	0
Running	95	5	0

*From Schutt RC, Fleck SJ: Production and utilization of energy in athletes. *Orthop Clin North Am* 1983; 14:459–467. Used by permission.

used. As contraction speed increases, force production decreases. Type I fibers, rich in mitochondria, myoglobin (which serves as an oxygen store), and oxidative enzymes, resist fatigue better than do Type II fibers. Type I fibers predominate in muscle active in antigravity activity and maintaining posture. These muscles are more resistant to fatigue than muscles used for brief intensive activity in which Type II fibers (with a predominance of glycolytic enzymes) are dominant. Muscles with a higher percentage of Type II fibers suffer more muscle strains.

II. The total fiber population of muscle is fixed and not influenced by training. Muscle fibers do enlarge, and, with increase in fiber size, more area of the muscle is occcupied by the trained fiber type. Biochemical alterations can occur, increasing aerobic capacity.

Changes are primarily due to selective hypertrophy of Type I fibers. It appears that the relative portion of subtypes of Type II fibers can be influenced by training (Table 5–3). Thus, the fatigue resistance of Type II fibers can be increased by endurance training.*

*In addition to specific cellular modifications, a physical conditioning program can also increase aerobic capacity by improving cardiac output and increasing hemoglobin level. On the whole, Type II fibers are more liable than Type I fibers to undergo work hypertrophy. The ultimate size of a muscle fiber is inversely proportional to its metabolic rate. The lower metabolic rate of Type II fibers allows them to more easily attain a larger diameter than Type I fibers with work.

TABLE 5–3.
Training Changes*

Anaerobic Training
  Increased lactic acid tolerance
  Increased ATP and CP
  Increased myocardial thickness
  Increased enzyme activity (phosphagen and
    anaerobic glycolysis systems)
Aerobic Training
  Increased fat and glycogen availability
  Increased oxidative capacity (fats and glycogen)
  Increased enzyme activity (oxidation of fats and
    glycogen)
  Increased ventricular volume
  Increased mitochondrial size and number
General Training
  Decreased total body fat
  Increased lean body mass
  Increased cardiovascular capacity
  Increased hemoglobin
  Increased blood volume
  Decreased blood pressure
  Increased heat acclimatization
  Decreased triglyceride and blood cholesterol levels

*From Schutt RC, Fleck SJ: Production and utilization of energy
in athletes. *Orthop Clin North Am* 1983; 14:459–467. Used by
permission.

After acute injury, muscles atrophy. Slow twitch muscle fibers atrophy first, presumably due to loss of the normal proprioception to which slow twitch fibers respond that occurs in the postural muscles. Even though slow twitch fibers atrophy first, fast twitch fibers also atrophy after injury. Pain is one of the inhibitors of fast twitch function.

BIBLIOGRAPHY

Dowben R: Contractility, with special reference to skeletal muscle, in Mount-castle V (ed): *Medical Physiology*, vol. 1. St Louis, CV Mosby Co, 1980.

Eisenberg BR, Brown JMC, Salmons S: Restoration of fast muscle characteristics following cessation of chronic stimulation. *Cell Tissue Res* 1984; 238: 221–230.

Gadian D, et al: Examination of a myopathy by phosphorus nuclear magnetic resonance. *Lancet* 1981; 10:774–775.

Griffiths RD, Cady EB, Edwards RHT, et al: Muscle energy metabolism in

Duchenne dystrophy studied by ^{31}P-NMR: Controlled trials show no effect of allopurinol or ribose. *Muscle Nerve* 1985; 8:760–767.

Margaria R: The sources of muscular energy. *Sci Am* 1972; 226:84–91.

Newsholme EA, Leech AR: *Biochemistry for the Medical Sciences.* New York, John Wiley & Sons, 1983, pp 146–158.

Ross BD, et al: Examination of a case of suspected McArdle's syndrome by ^{31}P nuclear magnetic resonance. *N Engl J Med* 1981; 304:1338–1342.

Schutt RC, Jr, Fleck SJ: Production and utilization of energy in athletes. *Orthop Clin North Am* 1983; 9:459–467.

Walton JN (ed): *Disorders of Voluntary Muscles,* ed 4. New York, Churchill Livingston, Inc, 1981.

Waters R, Hilsop H, Perry J, et al: Energetics, application to the study and management of locomotor disabilities. *Orthop Clin North Am* 1978; 9:351–356.

6

Mechanical Properties of Muscle

"A few observations and much reasoning leads to error; many observations and a little reasoning to truth."

Alexis Carrel (1873–1935)

The ultimate effect of a muscular contraction is produced by the interaction of several mechanical factors, including fiber direction, joint position, and location of insertion. As noted in the section on anatomy, where muscle fiber is oriented longitudinally, tension generated can contribute directly, through contraction, to total muscle tension produced. Pennate muscle fibers insert at an angle into longitudinally oriented connective tissue. This angular insertion prohibits rapid tension generation. However, the increased cross-sectional area of pennate muscles provides for greater available fiber tension.

Joint position and point of muscle attachment in relation to the center of movement of the joint are critical in the production of effective motion because they are determining factors in the generation of torque. Ideally, the most effective moment for any given plane of motion is produced when the angle of muscle insertion is at 90 degrees to the mobile segment of the joint. Additional compressive or distractive forces result at other angles of insertion. The length of the moment arm of the muscle varies throughout the range of motion of the joint moved. These factors, along with force-velocity and length-tension considerations, produce the ultimate moment for a given angle for any joint.

The properties of those tissues comprising the musculotendinous unit are also important to clinically applied muscle mechanics (Fig 6–1). The contractile component is composed of myosin and actin filaments. The elastic elements consist of the endomysium, epimysium, and perimysium. These tissues terminate by converging to form the tendon. The relationship of these components to each other is responsible for the mechanical properties of muscle. The contraction of muscle generates force. There are two types of contraction (Fig 6–2).

I. Isometric—where muscle length is held constant.
II. Isotonic—where muscle length changes in "constant tension."
    A. Concentric contracture—where a load is less than the isometric force a muscle can produce; the muscle shortens and lifts the load. Such contraction performs acceleratory motions, or positive work.
    B. Eccentric—where load is greater than the isometic force, the load elongates the actively contracting muscle, which resists this lengthening, performing decelerated, or negative, work. Muscle in eccentric contraction is seriously vulnerable to strain or rupture.

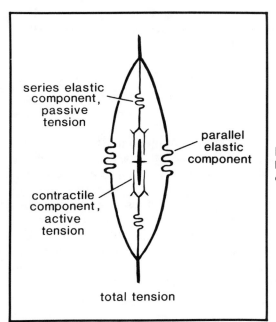

FIG 6–1.
Muscle model: functional components of striated muscle.

ISOTONIC CONTRACTION

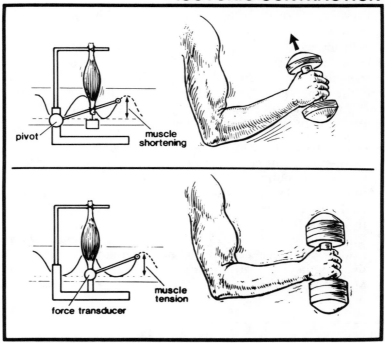

ISOMETRIC CONTRACTION

FIG 6–2.
Isotonic contraction *(top)* and isometric contraction *(bottom).*

Various exercise regimens that exploit force-tension properties of muscle are available. For instance, variable resistance machines provide exercise through a lever arm or cam arrangement that varies the amount of resistance offered in an attempt to match the strength curve of the individual. Isokinetic exercise can be provided at a constant velocity or speed where the resistance is not set. Isokinetic training increases strength to a greater extent than does isotonic training. Isokinetic training also causes greater increases in isometric strength. Motor performance is more improved by isotonic than by isometric training. Variable resistance may be superior to isotonic training, as far as increase in strength is concerned. Variable resistance also may increase motor performance to a greater extent than isometric training.

BIOELECTRIC RESPONSES OF MUSCLE

I. Summation of tension—where a second stimulus is applied to a muscle before the twitch elicited by the first stimulus subsides, a second contraction will be added to the response that is already in progress. Thus, relaxation is delayed and tension increases above that observed during the first twitch.

II. Tetanus—sustained muscular tension resulting from a volley of impulses (always greater than or equal to the tension generated during a single twitch).

    A. Summation of tension culminating in tetanus is achieved by increase of sarcoplasmic calcium concentration secondary to repeated action potentials (Fig 6–3). This activates more and more cross bridges, sites at which muscle tension is generated.

    B. Myofilament tension is transmitted through a series of elements (muscle cross bridges, sarcoplasm, sarcolemma, endomysium, myotendon junction, and tendon) possessing various degrees of elasticity. They act as a "spring" between the object upon which the muscle is acting and the muscular force. The "series elastic element" also has a major component in cross bridges.

III. Length-tension relationship. When a sarcomere is stretched to maximal length, there is no actin-myosin filament overlap (Fig 6–4). Thus, no tension can be generated. At shorter and shorter sarcomere lengths, the tension generated increases as there is more actin-myosin filament overlap. Maximum tension is reached at the point of maximal overlap. The classic length-tension

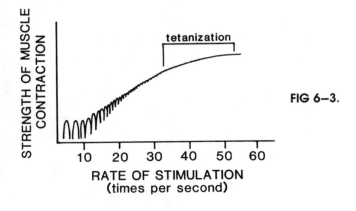

FIG 6–3.

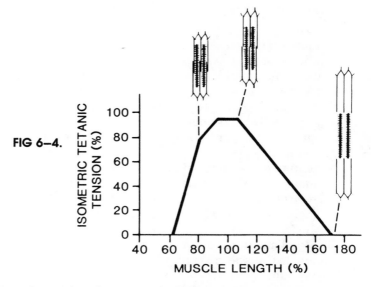

FIG 6–4.

(strength) relationship for a muscle fiber indicates that for a fixed length contraction there is an ideal length (resting length) at which maximum tension can be developed (Fig 6–5). At 75% of this length, the fiber can generate 75% of its power. At 60% of this length, we have zero force. If the fiber is lengthening during contraction, it will generate more force at each step in length than it can at the same length while fixed.

Clinical Relevance

Alterations of morphological, mechanical, and physiological features of muscle are important concerns in clinical management.

BLIX CURVE

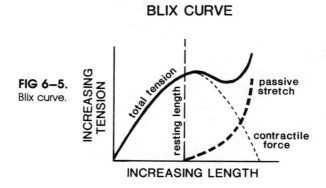

FIG 6–5.
Blix curve.

 I. Muscle lengthening may act as a shock absorber and lower the tensile stress on bone. Failures of muscle are not uncommon, and muscle rupture may result if the muscle is passively pulled beyond its ultimate tensile stress.
   A. Muscle rupture from simple stretch is usually rare in the absence of direct trauma.
   B. More common is complete muscle rupture due to forced stretching while the muscle is contracting or contracted (eccentric). This results from instant incoordination and is what usually happens when the biceps brachii, triceps surae, or quadriceps ruptures.
   C. Muscle tissue rupture is more common than tendon rupture as the maximum stress to failure for normal tendon is approximately twice that for normal muscle.
   D. Most strains and ruptures occur in two joint muscles. This is because tension is being generated to create movement or stabilization at one joint while stress is applied at the other.
 II. Precontraction stretching can effectively lengthen the elastic component and allow the production of tension either passively or with less contraction of active elements than is required for a shortening contraction.
   A. Eccentric contractions can also be used effectively to elicit muscle tension that may not be perceivable by patients performing a shortening contraction.
   B. Elastic energy can be transformed into kinetic energy by stretching muscle preceding contraction, thus using the elastic element to generate tension.
III. Success in muscle transfer depends in great measure on correct muscle length that considers the length-tension factors of muscle action. Excessive lengthening may remove the musculotendinous unit from the tension generating range.
IV. Shortening of muscle due to immobilization can result in subsequent limitation of extensibility because of shortening of the elastic element.
 V. The total number of sarcomeres decreases during immobilization in a shortened position. In adult muscle immobilized in a lengthened position, the number of sarcomeres increases, but not in very young muscles and not during recovery following immobilization in a shortened position.
VI. Atrophy of myofibrillar content follows muscle immobilization in the shortened position. After six weeks immobilization of an injured leg, the mean muscle fiber area decreases by approximately 25%.

VII. Time course of tension development is also clinically important. For instance, if tension does not develop to an appropriate level before heel strike during gait, the patient may not be able to maintain more proximal joints in the extended position during stance.

VIII. The body increases its energy efficiency by arranging for single muscles to activate two joints. Because fiber length in two-joint muscles is usually insufficient to permit cumulative movement in all the joints, the muscle passes over the joints in such a way that it is stretched at one joint while shortened at the other. For example, in analyzing hip and knee movements during running, if only one-joint muscles were available, a hip extensor would shorten (performing positive work) while a knee flexor would lengthen (dissipating energy). A hamstring muscle, following its normal stretch-shorten sequence, can perform both kinetic tasks with significant energy savings for the system.

IX. Physical therapy rehabilitation should be based on an understanding of the length-tension and force-velocity relationships of muscle.

BIBLIOGRAPHY

Albright JA, Brand RA: *The Scientific Basis of Orthopaedics.* New York, Appleton-Century-Crofts, 1979.

Elftman H: Biomechanics of muscle: Instructional course lectures. *Am Acad Orthop Surg* 1966; 48:363–377.

Huxley HE: Muscular contraction and cell motility. *Nature* 1973; 243:445–449.

Lehmkuhl DL: Local factors in muscle performance. Journal of the American Physical Therapy Association, *J Am Phys Ther Assoc* 1966; 46:473–485.

Pollack GH, Sugi H: *Contractile Mechanisms in Muscle.* New York, Plenum Publishing Corp, 1984, pp 453–541 and pp 737–797.

PART II

Clinical Techniques

7

Diagnosis of Neuromuscular Disease

"What is the hardest of all? That which you hold the most simple; seeing with your own eyes what is spread out before you."

Johann Wolfgang von Goethe (1749–1832)

"More is missed by not looking than by not knowing."

Thomas McCrae (1870–1935)

The diagnosis of muscle disease (Fig 7–1) is made on the basis of clinical history, physical examination, genetic evaluation, and special studies which include muscle enzymes, electromyography, and muscle biopsy.

HISTORY

A detailed history is taken. Generally speaking, the symptoms of neuromuscular disease are those of weakness. One must inquire into the duration of the symptom, what exacerbates or relieves it, whether it is constant or intermittent, progressing or diminishing, whether there are associated symptoms (such as pain), and the effect of medications on the weakness. Queries should also be directed toward:

53

Name_____Age____Occupation_____

Weight: Maximum weight with date_____Average weight_____
　　　　　Present weight____Weight loss or gain with duration_____

Birth and Developmental History:

　　　Movement in utero_____
　　　Length of Labor___Complications_____Birth weight____
　　　At risk factors (Rh., etc.)_____
　　　Convulsions_____Jaundice____O$_2$ lack at birth_____
Motor Milestones:
　　　Sitting_____Standing_____Walking_____
Symptoms:
　　　Stairs____Run____Rise____Falling____Jump_____
　　　Clumsiness____Rising from floor____Other_____
　　　Shoulder, arm, and hand function_____
　　　Description of gait (at onset of illness)_____
Family History:
　　　Father_____Mother_____Brothers and Sisters_____
　　　Cousins_____Other relations with possible m.d._____
Past Medical History:
　　　First symptom noted (age)_____saw M.D._____
　　　Original diagnosis_____
　　　Prescriptions (medication, bracing, P.T.)_____
　　　_____
　　　Progression_____
　　　Other significant illnesses_____
Other development:
　　　Intellectual_____Personality_____
Cranial Nerve and Thoracic Involvement:
　　　Facial musculature_____Dysphagia_____Dysarthria_____
　　　Breathing_____Frequency of respiratory infections_____
Development of Deformities:
　　　Lower extremities____Upper extremities____Spine_____
　　　_____
Cardiorespiratory:
　　　Palpitation____Dyspnea____Chest pain____Cyanosis_____
　　　Dependent edema_____Orthopnea_____Cough_____
Gastrointestinal:
　　　Eating habits_____Appetite_____Vomiting_____
　　　Nausea_____Pain or distress_____
　　　Bowel habits and control_____
Neurologic:
　　　Paresthesias_____Pain_____
　　　Muscle cramps_____Trophic changes_____

FIG 7–1.
A and **B,** muscle disease work-up check list.

General Examination:

B.P._____Pulse_____Respiration_____Temp._____
Nutrition and General Appearance_____
Head_____Neck_____Skin_____Heart_____
Lungs_____Chest_____Abdomen_____
Spine_____Extremities_____
Weakness and wasting_____Contractures_____
Facial and extra-ocular musculature_____
Neck musculature_____EENT_____
Neurologic findings: Cranial nerves_____Sensory_____
   Reflexes_____
   Babinski_____Hoffman_____Bell's sign_____
   Fasciculations_____Myotonia_____
Pseudohypertrophy_____Obesity_____
Cataracts_____Baldness_____Fever_____
Rash_____Tenderness_____
Performance:
   Run_____Jump_____Rise_____Gait_____
   Other_____
   Miscellaneous_____

Laboratory Work-Up:

Enzymes_____Biopsy_____
EMG_____EKG_____
Other_____
Physical Therapy_____Occupational Therapy_____
X-Rays_____
_____

Social work-up_____
Psychologist_____Dietician_____
Other medical consultations_____

Summary of Significant Findings:
_____
_____
_____

Impression:
_____
_____
_____

Plan for further work-up and treatment:
_____
_____
_____

I. Timing of motor milestones—often delayed (50% of DMD fail to walk until 18 months).
II. Abnormalities in gait.
III. Evidence of hypotonia during infancy.
IV. Cramps and stiffness (Table 7–1).
V. Pregnancy and birth—usually normal except that some mothers report diminished fetal movements.
VI. Motor, language, and adaptive social behavior.
VII. A detailed family history of similar disease.
VIII. Exposure to extrinsic causes of muscle weakness, such as organic and inorganic toxins, trauma, infections, drugs, or other such agents.

PHYSICAL EXAMINATION

A complete physical examination is performed with particular attention paid to:

I. Gait—look for waddling and equinus.
II. Posture—evaluate balance, lordosis, and postural base.
III. Facies—inspect movements, expression, wasting, atrophy, and look for fasciculations.
IV. Early signs of Duchenne muscular dystrophy.
 A. Flat feet (secondary to heel cord contracture).
 B. Weak shoulder extension.
 C. Hesitance when ascending stairs.
 D. Slight lateral pelvic shift when arising from seated position on floor.

TABLE 7–1.
Causes of Muscle Cramps*

I. At rest. Usually normal.
II. Exertional. Relieved by rest. May be associated myoglobinuria.
 A. Benign and low-grade muscular dystrophy (limb girdle or Becker types).
 B. Metabolic disorders.
  1. Glycogenoses
   a) Type V (phosphorylase deficiency).
   b) Type VII (phosphofructokinase deficiency).
  2. Lipid metabolism disorders
   a) Carnitine palmityl transferase deficiency.
 C. Other myoglobinuric syndromes.

*From Dubowitz V: *Muscle Disorders in Childhood.* Philadelphia, WB Saunders Co., 1978. Used by permission.

    E. Acceleration during final stage of sitting down.

    F. Poor standing jump.

    G. Waddling run.

V. Later signs of Duchenne muscular dystrophy.

    A. Waddling gait.

    B. Frequent falling.

    C. Difficulty ascending stairs.

    D. Slipping through at the shoulders.

    E. Positive Gowers' sign (Fig 7–2).

    F. Lordosis.

    G. Progressive equinus.

    H. Calf hypertrophy.

    I. Weak neck flexion.

    J. Depression of deep tendon reflexes, except those of Achilles tendons.

VI. In evaluating infants, note coordination during play and examine

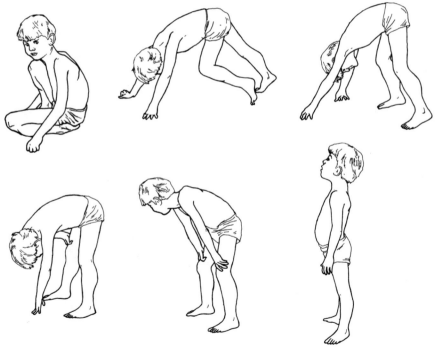

FIG 7–2.
Gower's (Tripod) sign.

for key motor milestones (Table 7–2). Observe and palpate for muscle hypertrophy. Consistency of a muscle with "pseudohypertrophy" in DMD is rubbery and firm, as contrasted with the flabby feeling of an atrophied muscle or the firm resilience of a normal one.

Examine infants for head lag (floppiness). Evaluate for hypotonia. Test range of motion of all major joints for contracture. Percuss muscles for myotonia or myoedema (hypothyroidism). Quantitatively assess key muscle groups, but note that on a grading system of 0–5, almost 45% loss is required to drop the grade from 5 to 4 in a large postural muscle group. Also remember that there is no individual muscle action. Each muscle has agonists, synergists, and fixators, as well as antagonists.

It is unnecessary to evaluate every muscle or even every muscle group in the body. Quantitative strength assessment should be made

TABLE 7–2.
Some Motor Milestones in Normal Development (Average)*

Birth
  Flexor posture of limbs, able to sustain head in line with body in ventral suspension and supine.
3 months
  Momentary sitting posture, flexed forward.
6 months
  Sits leaning forward on hands. Lifts head spontaneously when supine. Takes weight on legs well.
9 months
  Sits. Pivots. Pulls to standing position.
1 year
  Walks with help. Cruises.
15 months
  Walks unaided. Creeps up stairs.
18 months
  Walks without falling. Runs. Climbs stairs unaided.
2 years
  Able to run well. Kicks a ball. Goes up and down stairs.
3 years
  Stands on one leg. Jumps off a step.
4 years
  Hops on one foot (just).
5 years
  Good ability to hop on either leg.

*From Dubowitz V: *Muscle Disorders in Childhood.* Philadelphia, WB Saunders Co, 1978. Used by permission.

of major postural muscle groups, those of the shoulders, hips, knees and ankles.

Deep tendon reflexes disappear as muscle strength and spindle function decrease. The Achilles deep tendon reflexes persist because the triceps surae tendon is the strongest in the body and takes a direct course from origin to insertion. The dominant Achilles is the last deep tendon reflex to be lost. One should look for fasciculations (they can sometimes be auscultated), particularly in the tongue (a skinned muscle), and also the fine tremor (minipolymyoclonus) seen in SMA. This fingertip tremor is regular, in contrast to tremors secondary to other neurological disease. The spine should be inspected for scoliosis. This is sometimes obvious with one hip and shoulder higher than the other. Minimal curves can often be demonstrated by sighting down the spine with the patient bending forward from the waist. Rotation is emphasized in this position as one side of the back stands higher than the other (Table 7–3).

In general, myopathies show proximal (limb-girdle) weakness, whereas neuropathies begin distally. As a rule, weakness exceeds atrophy in myopathies, whereas atrophy exceeds weakness in neuropathic disease (Table 7–4).

TABLE 7–3.
Evaluation Checklist

Weakness
    Age of onset
    Rapidity of onset
    Static or progressive
    Distribution
Pain
    Exertional
    At rest
    Type (dull, cramping, etc.)
Fasciculations
    Myokymia
Hypertrophy (pseudohypertrophy of muscle)
    Location
Myotonia
    Effort or percussion
Atrophy
    Distribution (focal or diffuse)
Contractures
Fatigability
Tone
    Palpation of muscle
Deep tendon reflexes

TABLE 7–4.
Myopathy and Neuropathy

CATEGORY	MYOPATHY	NEUROPATHY
Muscle involvement	Usually proximal muscles	Muscles are affected in distribution of root and nerves; when diffuse, involvement is usually more distal
Atrophy	More proximal	More peripheral in distribution
Fasciculations	None	+
Deep tendon reflexes	Present; they are lost when myopathy is end stage	Lost early

DIFFERENTIAL MUSCULAR WEAKNESS

Most myopathies have the same pathokinetics of progressive muscle weakness. Differences lie in the rapidity of progression and degree of weakness and contracture (Table 7–5). For example:

I. Neck extensors, toe flexors and tibialis posterior are commonly spared in all types of myopathy. However, all groups show some involvement of lower and middle trapezii.

II. In DMD, anterior neck flexors (particularly sternocleidomastoid) are involved late in the disease. They are, however, involved more frequently than in other myopathies. Weak neck flexion is an "early sign" in myositis.

TABLE 7–5.
Patterns of Muscle Weakness and Sparing in Early Muscular Dystrophy

	NECK AND UPPER EXTREMITY		TRUNK AND LOWER EXTREMITY	
PATTERN	INVOLVED	SPARED	INVOLVED	SPARED
Common in all groups	Lower trapezius Middle trapezius	Neck extensors		Gastrocnemius Tibialis posterior Toe flexors
Common in Duchenne and limb-girdle	Rhomboids Latissimus dorsi Inward rotators	Upper trapezius Biceps Triceps	Gluteus maximus Hip adductors	
Unique patterns				
Duchenne	Anterior neck flexors (SCM)		Anterior abdominals Gluteus medius Tensor fasciae latae Iliopsoas	Hamstrings
Limb-girdle		Brachioradialis		
Fascioscapulohumeral	Upper pectoralis major	Lower pectoralis major	Tibialis anterior	Back extensors Iliopsoas Gluteus medius Tensor fasciae latae Quadriceps

III. Hamstring strength is often preserved in DMD (lateral hamstrings spared the longest).

IV. Brachioradialis is commonly strong in LGD.

V. In FSH, lower pectoralis major is often spared, although tibialis anticus is frequently involved early in the disease.

VI. In LGD, there may be selective absence of a single muscle. This is also noted in some of the morphologically specific myopathies (e.g., central core disease).

VII. In all the common dystrophies, the pattern of loss is from proximal to distal. DMD and LGD are symmetrical in distribution, whereas FSH and Becker's dystrophy may be asymmetrical. Flexors are usually weaker than extensors in the trunk and neck. Extensors are usually weaker than flexors in the hips and shoulders. However, triceps brachii may be stronger than biceps brachii in Becker's dystrophy.

VIII. One of the earliest signs of FSH (even in forme fruste cases) may be finger, wrist, or toe extensor weakness.

IX. Hip abductors are weakened more frequently in myopathy than in neuropathy. With weakened hip abduction, loss of the shock absorber function of the hip abductors results in an antalgic gait characterized by a thud on foot placement.

X. In LGD, the shoulder lacks fixation and tends to fall forward. This, associated with atrophy of the sternal head of pectoralis major, results in an accentuation of the anterior axillary line. Patients with advanced LGD walk with the arms held loosely at their sides with the dorsum of the hands and forearms pointing forward. They "throw" their shoulders due to weakness of shoulder protraction. With proximal limb-girdle weakening, the upper arm atrophies, giving a "Popeye" appearance to the normal forearm.

XI. Dorsiflexor weakness in FSH and late DMD may lead to the "praying mantis" position of the flexed wrist and fingers.

Clinical Signs Indicating Muscle Weakness

I. Head and neck.
A. Ptosis.
1. Retroflexion of the neck in order to see straight ahead.
2. Particularly seen in myasthenia gravis.
B. Weakness of extraocular muscles.
1. Especially in oculopharyngeal muscular dystrophy.
C. Masseter muscle weakness.

      1. Jaw may open spontaneously.
  D. Temporalis muscle wasting—hollowing at the temples—seen in dystrophia myotonica.
  E. Facial muscle weakness.
      1. Patients cannot whistle, blow up a balloon, or suck through a straw—seen in FSH.
      2. Absence of normal movement of facial muscles in response to emotion.
      3. Loss of nasolabial folds and other normal facial wrinkles, seen in FSH.
      4. Difficulty with speech (particularly labials), seen in FSH.
  F. Difficulty with swallowing.
      1. Found in pseudobulbar palsy as well as myositis.
  G. Palatal weakness.
      1. Lower motor neuron lesions involving the palate result in a voice that has an echoing nasal quality. The vowels are hollow; the consonants, particularly hard C, are difficult to pronounce.
      2. Spastic speech (pseudobulbar palsy) has a forced quality.
      3. Scanning speech (cerebellar disease)—disjointed.
      4. Laryngeal weakness. May result in hoarseness, and the glottal stop is lost.
  H. Neck weakness.
      1. Flexor weakness (late in DMD—early in myositis).
      2. Wasting of sternocleidomastoid (clavicular before sternal head).
   I. Tongue wasting, resulting in wrinkled or scalloped lateral borders.
II. Shoulders.
  A. Prominence more noticeable.
      1. Scapular winging (particularly in FSH).
      2. High "trapezius hump"—especially prominent during abduction of arms.
  B. Throwing motion necessary for forward elevation of arm.
III. Hands.
  A. Wasting of major muscle groups, including "guttering" of interosseous muscles.
  B. Simian hand—noted in lesions of median nerve.
  C. Claw hand—seen in lesions of ulnar nerve.
  D. Extensor weakness (wrist-fingers)—radial nerve lesions.
IV. Hip.
  A. Hip extensor weakness, accompanied by hip flexion contracture, leading to increased lumbar lordosis.

    B. Inability to jump, rise from a seated position, or easily descend stairs.

V. Knee.

    A. Quadriceps weakness evident in tripod sign (Gowers) on arising from the floor or a seated position.

    B. Weakness of vastus medialis (which produces final 10 degrees of knee extension), causing extension instability.

    C. More difficulty descending than ascending stairs (the knee is loaded with up to seven times body weight when descending stairs).

VI. Leg.

    A. Where anterior tibial and peroneal groups are atrophied, tibia assumes a sharpened configuration due to prominence of its anterior border.

VII. Ankle.

    A. Evertor and dorsiflexor weakness may lead to frequent ankle sprains.

    B. Foot drop due to either myopathy or neuropathy.

        1. Extensor digitorum brevis may be secondarily hypertrophied.

        2. Slapping-type gait with difficulty in plantar flexion from calf muscle weakness.

An examination of muscular strength should note evidence of hysterical weakness (by observing whether the patient moves the limb when unaware of being studied). Suspected hysterics can activate antagonist muscles, which should be palpated while testing muscle strength. In hysterical ptosis, the lower lid is always contracted.

Testing a patient's functional abilities in performing a standard set of tasks, such as stepping up, climbing, arising from a chair, etc., provides an excellent evaluation of the state of disability. The method utilized, as well as the time taken to perform the task, should be recorded. The activities most usefully assessed because they most frequently show abnormalities are arising from a seated position on the floor, stepping onto an elevation, arising from a chair, hopping on the toes, walking on the heels, and raising the arms overhead.

BIBLIOGRAPHY

Brooke M: *A Clinician's View of Neuromuscular Diseases*, ed 2. Baltimore, Williams & Wilkins Co, 1985.
Dubowitz V: *Muscle Disorders in Children.* Philadelphia, WB Saunders Co, 1978.

Rowland LP: Pathogenesis of muscular dystrophies. *Arch Neurol* 1976; 33:315–320.

Swash M, Schwartz M: *Neuromuscular Diseases*. New York, Springer-Verlag, 1981.

Walton J (ed): *Disorders of Voluntary Muscle,* ed 4. New York, Churchill Livingstone, Inc, 1981.

8

Serum Enzymes

"Nature is the great experimenter."
Anonymous

I. Normal muscle utilizes creatine and secretes creatinine.
II. In muscular dystrophy (as well as neuropathy), the reverse is true. There is a decreased urinary output of creatinine and an increase in the urine creatine level during the symptomatic stages of the disease. Also noted is a lower creatine tolerance because total muscle mass is decreased. The cause of creatinuria in myopathy is the inability of muscle to hold creatine. In neuropathy, the muscle cell cannot absorb the creatine, hence creatinuria.

Blood levels of serum aldolase, serum glutamic oxaloacetic transaminase (SGOT), serum glutamic pyruvic transaminase (SGPT), and lactic dehydrogenase (LDH) can all be increased in muscle disease (though elevation is not specific for myopathy). Serum pyruvate kinase is also increased in DMD, DMD carriers, and FSH.

CREATINE PHOSPHOKINASE: CPK (CREATINE KINASE: CK)

I. Provides the most sensitive biochemical index for the diagnosis of muscle disease.

A. Does not appear to increase in hepatic disease.
B. Very little contained in erythrocytes; thus hemolysis does not contaminate analysis.
C. Found in heart and brain.

II. Function. Reversibly catalyzes the transfer of an energy-rich bond from creatine phosphate to adenosine diphosphate (ADP), forming creatine and adenosine triphosphate (ATP) (Fig 8–1).

III. Isozymes. There are three isoenzymes of CPK: (1) BB (brain type), (2) MB (hybrid type), and (3) MM (muscle type). Both MB and MM ratios are changed in myopathy. Injured muscle tends to produce MB as it regenerates. LDH can be fractioned into five isozymes. It has been claimed that probands as well as DMD carriers show an increase in bands one and two, with a concomitant decrease in bands three, four and five of the LDH electrophoretic fractionation.

IV. Diagnosis of myopathy is commonly based on clinical findings, but enzyme determinations can:
A. Usually confirm the diagnosis (often before clinical findings are evident).
B. Often distinguish between a myopathy and a neuropathy. (Although serum enzymes may be elevated with muscular weakness of neurogenic origin, particularly in chronic denervating diseases, such elevation is usually not as high as that found in a myopathy.)
C. Occasionally differentiate certain primary myopathies from each other and from polymyositis.
D. Frequently detect a heterogenous, clinically healthy carrier of the sex-linked disease.
E. Follow the evolution and course of the myopathies (particularly the inflammatory variety), thus helping to evaluate therapy and providing an index for prognosis.

V. Serum CPK is increased in myopathy.
A. Highest in preclinical Duchenne muscular dystrophy.
1. Elevated in normal newborn because of birth trauma; falls to normal level by 4–7 days postdelivery.

FIG 8–1.

$$\text{Phosphocreatine} + \text{ADP} \xrightleftharpoons{\text{CPK}} \text{ATP} + \text{Creatine}$$

2. False negative can occur with examination of fetal blood drawn from umbilical vein; therefore, this method is unreliable.
B. Elevated in approximately 70%–80% of Duchenne carriers.
   1. The earlier the test is performed, the better the chance of an accurate result.
C. Modestly increased in limb-girdle dystrophy, FSH, and dystrophia myotonica.
D. Level cannot correlate well with duration of illness because CPK elevation and magnitude of its variations are proportional to remaining mass of dystrophic muscle and severity of disease. Thus, serum enzyme elevations are higher in early than in late DMD (approaching normal levels in the preterminal case), less striking in limb-girdle dystrophy and FSH, and least prominent in myotonic disease.
E. In polymyositis, degree of elevation depends on rate of progression, degree of weakness, and severity of inflammation. Elevated level of MB isoenzyme indicates muscle regeneration, not necessarily active myocarditis.
   1. Serial CPK determinations can be used to monitor effectiveness of steroid therapy in polymyositis. Decline of serum enzyme level anticipates clinical improvement by approximately three to six weeks. Conversely, a rise in enzyme level presages a decrease in muscle strength with about the same time lag.
VI. Range of CPK.
A. Higher in younger individuals, elevated in healthy teenage boys.
B. Higher in blacks than in whites.
C. Higher after exercise; less elevation in trained athletes. Higher in men after exercise.
D. Decreased in pregnancy.* Uninfluenced by oral contraceptives.
E. Can be normal or decreased in patients with certain connective tissue diseases (systemic lupus erythematosus, rheumatoid arthritis, Sjögren's syndrome).
F. Higher in outpatients than inpatients.
G. Higher in males than females.
H. Highest between ages 10–19 and 40–49. Increases with menopause.

*In contrast, pyruvate kinase activity does not seem to be influenced by pregnancy.

TABLE 8–1.
CPK Elevations, Signs, Symptoms, and Other Findings in Diseases With Muscle Weakness*

DISEASE	CPK	FAMILY HISTORY	PSEUDOHYPERTROPHY	REMISSION OR NONPROGRESSION	FASCICULATION AND FIBRILLATION
Duchenne muscular dystrophy					
Early in course	++++	++++	++++	0	±
Late in course	++	++++	++	0	0
Late onset variant	++++	++++	++++	0	±
Limb-girdle muscular dystrophy					
Early onset	++	+	0	0	0
Late onset	+	++	0	0	0
Fascioscapulohumeral dystrophy	+	+++	+	0	0
Myotonic dystrophy	±	+++	0	0	Myotonia
Acute myositis	+++	0	0	++++	+
Polymyositis	++	+	+	++	+
Benign muscular hypotonia	Normal	+	0	+++	0
Thyrotoxic myopathies	±	0	0	++	0
Spinal muscular atrophy	±	+	0	0	++++
Peripheral polyneuropathies	±	0	0	++	++
Amyotrophic lateral sclerosis	Normal	0	0	0	Fasciculations

*Adapted from Coodley EL (ed): *Diagnostic Enzymology.* Philadelphia, Lea & Febiger, p 263.

      I. Higher in the evening. Decreases January to June, increases by approximately 20% from July to December (circadian rhythm) in carriers of DMD.

VII. Conditions other than neuromuscular diseases in which CPK can be elevated include:

    A. Myocardial infarction.

    B. Intramuscular injection—usually returns to normal within one week.

    C. Alcoholism.

    D. Muscular injury.

    E. Malignant hyperthermia.

    F. Stroke, subarachnoid hemorrhage.

    G. Brain tumor.

    H. Convulsions—prolonged coma.

    I. Meningitis.

    J. Encephalitis.

    K. Acute psychosis.

    L. Hypokalemia (diuretic-, licorice-, or laxative-induced)

    M. A variety of acute abdominal conditions, including hemorrhagic pancreatitis, gangrene of the gallbladder, pancreatic CA.

    N. Untreated hypothyroidism.

    O. Acute pneumonitis.

    P. Eclampsia.

    Q. Electric countershock.

    R. Urologic procedures (cystoscopy, bladder biopsy).

    S. Radiotherapy.

    T. Sleep deprivation.

    U. Dissecting aneurysm.

    V. McLeod's syndrome (rare disorder characterized by weak expression of Kell antigens on red blood cells).

    Table 8–1 tabulates relative elevations of serum CPK enzyme activity correlated with other significant diagnostic parameters in a variety of neuromuscular diseases.

BIBLIOGRAPHY

Bourne GH: *The Structure and Function of Muscle,* ed 2. New York, Academic Press, 1972.

Coodley EL (ed): *Diagnostic Enzymology.* Philadelphia, Lea & Febiger, 1970.

Goto I: Creatine phosphokinase isozymes in neuromuscular disorders. *Arch Neurol* 1974; 31:116–119.

Hooshmand H, Dove J, Suter C: LDH isoenzymes in muscle diseases. *Neurology* (Minneapolis) 1969; 19:26–31.

Munsat TL, Baloh R, Pearson CM, et al: Serum enzyme alterations in neuromuscular disorders. *JAMA* 1973; 226:1536–1543.

Murphy EG: *The Chemistry and Therapy of Disorders of Voluntary Muscles.* Springfield, Illinois, Charles C Thomas, Publisher, 1964.

Nevins MA, Saran M, Bright M, et al: Pitfalls in interpreting serum creatine phosphokinase activity. *JAMA* 1973; 224:1382–1387.

Shumate JB, Brooke M, Carroll JE, et al: Increased serum creatine kinase after exercise: A sex-linked phenomenon. *Neurology* 1979; 29:902–904.

Takahashi K, Shutta K, Matsuo B, et al: Serum creatine kinase isoenzymes in Duchenne muscular dystrophy. *Clin Chim Acta* 1977; 75:435–552.

Telford IW: *Experimental Muscular Dystrophies in Animals: A Comparative Study.* Springfield, Illinois, Charles C Thomas, Publisher, 1971.

Yasminey WG, Ibrahim GA, Abbasnezhad M, et al: Isoenzyme distribution of creatine kinase and lactate dehydrogenase in serum and skeletal muscle in Duchenne muscular dystrophy, collagen disease, and other muscular disorders. *Clin Chem* 1978; 24:1985–1989.

Zellweger J, Antonik A: Newborn screening for Duchenne muscular dystrophy. Muscular Dystrophy Associations of America, Inc, National Institutes of Health, USPHS Clinical Research Center, Grant MO1 FR 59, and state services for crippled children special project budget MR 12.

9

Electrophysiology

"I think that I shall always see, a motor unit as a tree."

Anonymous

EMG

Electrodiagnostic techniques can usually delineate that segment of the motor unit involved by a disease process. Anterior horn cell, nerve root, peripheral nerve, and neuromuscular junction of skeletal muscle fiber may be distinguished. The following cautions are advised:

I. Select appropriate muscles for examination (proximal in suspect myopathy, distal in suspect neuropathy).
II. Do not draw muscle enzymes immediately after an EMG because the exam may give a false positive.
III. Do not biopsy a recently needled muscle because the exam produces needle artifacts.

Important components of the EMG include:

I. Amplitude.
II. Frequency.
III. Duration of the summed action potentials.

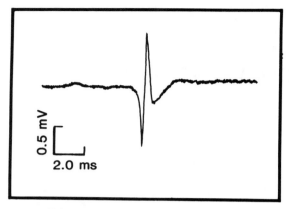

FIG 9–1.
Normal human motor unit configuration.

Characteristics of the EMG:

I. Normal (Fig 9–1).
  A. Silent at rest.
  B. Occasional myokymia is not abnormal.
  C. Generation of normal triphasic motor unit potentials with activity.
  D. Interference pattern on summation with increased activity.
II. Denervation.
  A. Frequent fibrillation potentials (Fig 9–2). However, fibrillation potentials can occur in myopathy because of muscle fiber necrosis and secondary terminal nerve involvement from connective tissue changes, especially in inflammatory myositis (polymyositis-dermatomyositis).
  B. Positive sharp waves. Like fibrillation potentials, they probably originate from single-muscle fibers, occur more commonly in peripheral nerve disorders than in more proximal lesions, and are more prominent in acute denervating diseases.
  C. Fasciculation potentials (Fig 9–3). High-amplitude polyphasic

FIG 9–2.
Fibrillations.

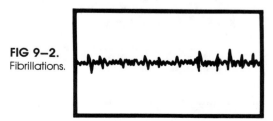

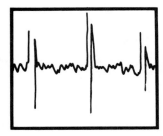

FIG 9–3.
Irregular, spontaneous fasciculations.

potentials of long duration, which occur at rest and are produced mainly by lesions of the anterior horn cell.
D. Group polyphasic potentials (Fig 9–4). Muscle action poten-
tials with more than four phases, occurring as groups.
E. Reduced interference pattern or increased amplitude of muscle
potential; due to reinnervation of muscle fibers by the sprout-
ing of uninvolved nerve cell processes.
F. Increased duration of muscle action potential.
G. Decreased frequency of muscle action potential, because fewer
units are available for firing, having atrophied secondary to
disease of the motor neuron.
III. Myopathy.
A. Increased insertional activity.
B. Short duration polyphasic potentials.
C. Retained interference pattern.
D. Reduced amplitude of muscle action potential, because scat-
tered fibers within the sampled field are not functioning.
E. Reduced duration of muscle action potential.
F. Increased frequency of muscle action potential, because more
units are called upon to support muscle contraction (Fig 9–5).
G. It is claimed by some that the presence of a short-duration, re-

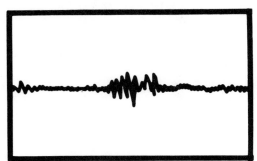

FIG 9–4.
Polyphasic pattern.

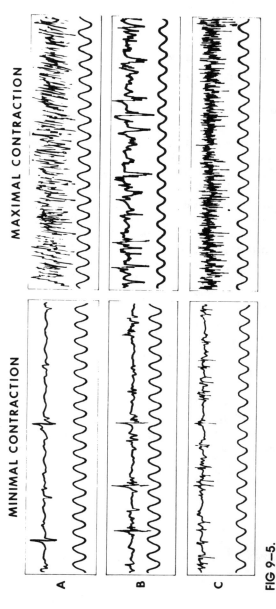

FIG 9–5.
EMG in *(A)* normal, *(B)* neuropathic, and *(C)* myopathic muscle. (Modified from Walton JN (ed): *Disorders of Voluntary Muscle*, ed 3. New York, Churchill Livingstone, Inc, 1974.

duced-amplitude, increased-frequency motor unit potential may be seen in any neurogenic disorder causing fractionation of the motor unit and is not therefore conclusive evidence of myopathy.

NOTE: Some of the morphologically specific myopathies, such as nemaline myopathy and central core disease, usually have a normal EMG. McArdle's disease (phosphorylase deficiency) demonstrates electrical silence when muscle contraction persists. Pompe's disease (Type II glycogen storage disease) shows profuse hyperirritability of the muscle cell membrane, with positive waves and fibrillation potentials.

IV. Myotonia (Fig 9–6).
    A. Trains of spiked potentials and positive waves fired at a high frequency, which then wax and wane until they die out (the dive bomber effect).
    B. Pseudomyotonia (a term applied to bursts of myotonic activity seen in neuromuscular disorders without clinical myotonia, such as Type II glycogenosis).
    Figure 9–7 is a diagram of typical EMG responses.
V. Polymyositis.
    A. A combination of neuropathic and myopathic features, including:
        1. Prolonged insertional activity.
        2. Short-duration action potentials.
        3. Positive sharp waves.
        4. A complex polyphasic electrical pattern with greatly reduced amplitude of voluntary muscular contraction.
        5. Spontaneous fibrillation potentials, occurring at complete rest or after mild mechanical muscular stimulation.
        6. Groups of repetitive potentials of brief duration.

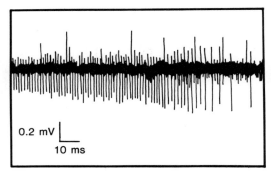

0.2 mV

10 ms

FIG 9–6.
Myotonic discharge.

NORMAL

MYOPATHY

NEUROPATHY

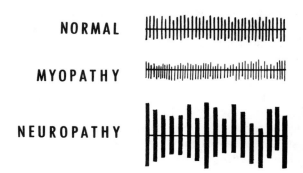

FIG 9–7.
Schematic diagram of features of electrical response in EMG for *normal, myopathic* (increased frequency, decreased duration, decreased amplitude), and *neuropathic* (decreased frequency, increased duration, increased amplitude) states. (Modified from Vick NA: *Chicago Medicine* 1973; August 11.)

    B. Special electrodiagnostic techniques.
        1. Late response studies (H and F reflexes) are used for evaluating the function of the most proximal segments of the peripheral nerves.
        2. The blink reflex is useful in evaluating patients with Bell's palsy, multiple sclerosis, and other brain stem and cranial nerve disorders.
        3. Single fiber EMG offers a more sensitive and sophisticated diagnostic evaluation for diseases of the neuromuscular junction.
        4. Quantitative motor-unit analysis permits statistical projections concerning the likelihood of a motor unit disease being present.
        5. Cortical-evoked potential studies. Evaluate spinal cord injury and functional recovery following head trauma.
 VI. Nerve Conduction Velocity.
    A. Types.
        1. Motor velocity is reduced in peripheral neuropathies:
            a) Slight decrease (or normal) in axonal disease.
            b) Marked depression with segmental demyelinization.
            c) Normal in myopathies and muscular atrophies.
        2. Sensory velocity (useful in evaluating conditions such as peroneal muscular atrophy or Friedreich's ataxia, where it is reduced).

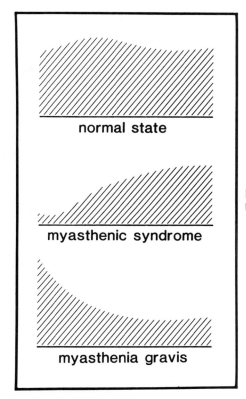

FIG 9–8.
Evoked muscle potential.

B. Repetitive nerve stimulation (evoked muscle potentials) (Fig 9–8).
   1. Produces characteristic patterns (decremental or incremental) of muscle response in different diseases of the myoneural junction (e.g., myasthenia gravis, Eton-Lambert syndrome, etc.).

BIBLIOGRAPHY

Bender LF: Diagnostic electromyography. *JAMA* 1967; 199:137–141.

Campbell EDR: Electrodiagnosis in muscle disease. *Practitioner* 1976; 216: 414–419.

Kaplan J: Electromyography and nerve conduction velocities. *Curr Concepts Pain.* 1983; 1:11–16.

Samaha FJ: Medical intelligence: Current concepts, electrodiagnostic studies in neuromuscular disease. *N Engl J Med* 1971; 285:1344–1347.

Swaiman KL, Wright FS: *Neuromuscular Diseases of Infancy and Childhood.* Springfield, Illinois, Charles C Thomas, Publisher, 1970.

Vick NA: Disease of skeletal muscle—Current ideas of diagnosis and management. *Chicago Med* 1973; 76:621–625.

Warmolts JR, Engel WK: A critique of the "myopathic" electromyogram. *Trans Am Neurol Assoc* 1970; 95:173–177.

10

Muscle Biopsy

"Pathology is the accomplished tragedy, physiology the basis on which our treatment rests."

Edward Martin (1859–1938)

Muscle biopsy is an essential part of the workup of a suspected neuromuscular disorder. It may be the best way to arrive at a definitive diagnosis and accurate classification of the disease.

I. Technique.
  A. Muscle should be selected that is not so severely affected that it is largely replaced by connective tissue and fat. In early disease, choose a weak muscle, in late disease a strong one; a muscle graded 2 to 3 (poor to fair) is best.
    1. In most proximal disorders, the lateral quadriceps or biceps brachii are preferred because these muscles have an almost equal ratio of Type I to Type II fibers. Deltoid and soleus, on the other hand, may have a 60%–80% Type I predominance, and gastrocnemius may show a Type II predominance.
  B. If local anesthesia is used, do not traumatize the muscle under biopsy by the needle or by infiltration of muscle tissue with the anesthetic agent. Avoid epinephrine as it depletes

glycogen from muscle fibers and exhausts phosphorylase activity. Also avoid muscle recently needled for EMG. Never biopsy at the musculotendinous junction.
C. Open or needle biopsy technique may be employed (Fig 10–1).
D. A well-performed and expertly interpreted biopsy can usually distinguish a neuropathy from a myopathy, often diagnose an inflammatory myopathy, and frequently differentiate the morphologically specific myopathies.
E. Muscle biopsy can sometimes be used for purposes of determining prognosis, assessing degree of involvement, or evaluating therapy (i.e., in polymyositis). It is impossible by standard biopsy alone to categorically distinguish between the common muscular dystrophies (Duchenne, limb-girdle, FSH, dystrophia myotonica).
II. Staining (Fig 10–2).
   A variety of routine stains are employed. Histological stains include:
A. H & E, Gomori-trichrome, and Verhoeff-van Gieson for histological pattern, architecture, connective tissue, and vascular status. Degenerative/regenerative processes can also be demonstrated.
B. PAS, for glycogen content.
C. Oil red O or sudan black B, for lipid.
The histochemical stains include:
A. Myofibrillar ATPase (pH 9.4 or 4.6)-fiber type classification.
B. NADH-TR—oxidative activity, structural abnormality, mitochondrial changes.
Special stains:
A. RNA stain and acid phosphatase stains for focal degenerative/regenerative changes.

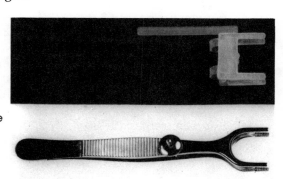

FIG 10–1.
Two types of muscle biopsy clamps designed to keep the specimen at its original in situ length. The one pictured above is made of disposable plastic.

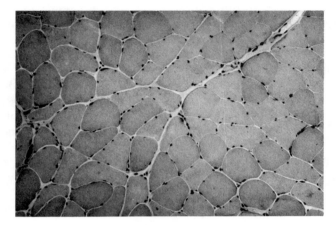

FIG 10–2.
Normal muscle.

B. Phosphorylase. In Type V glycogenosis, this enzyme is lacking.

C. Various chemical markers (antibodies, fluorescent dyes, radioactive labelled metabolites) and accompanying techniques (cytochemistry, immunochemistry, autoradiography, fluorescence microscopy) can be used to display muscle cell structure.

III. Histological changes noted in neuromuscular pathology.*
   A. Degeneration/necrosis/regeneration.
   B. Selective fiber type loss or other fiber type change.
   C. Fat and connective tissue replacement.
   D. Inflammatory cell infiltration.
   E. Nuclear abnormalities.
   F. Mitochondrial abnormalities.
   G. Excessive lipid or carbohydrate.
   H. Morphologically specific architectural changes.
   I. Fiber size variation, splitting, and internal nucleation, which are evidence of repeated cycles of necrosis and regeneration.

NOTE: Changes are usually diffuse in myopathy and scattered in neuropathy with adjacent normal tissue.

IV. Fiber type specific diseases: Differences in fiber type morphology.
   A. Changes in fiber size (Type I is normally slightly smaller than Type II).

*It has been suggested that agents that might protect against cellular damage occurring in myopathy include (1) calcium antagonists, (2) phospholipase inhibitors, and (3) antioxidants.

B. Fiber type predominance.
  1. Generally, Type I predominance is found in myopathies, particularly nemaline myopathy and DMD.
  2. Type II predominance is present in ALS.
C. Fiber type atrophy.
  1. Type II atrophy common in disuse atrophy, myasthenia gravis, steroid myopathy.
  2. Type I atrophy found in myotonic dystrophy, myotubular myopathy, congenital muscle fiber type disproportion, glycogenosis II and III.
D. Fiber hypertrophy.
  1. Type I hypertrophy seen in long-standing neurogenic disorders.
  2. Type II hypertrophy occurs in motor neuron disease.
E. Fiber type grouping.
  1. Found in neurogenic disorders.
V. Degenerative changes in muscle.
  A. Necrotic fibers.
  B. Fiber splitting.
  C. Central nucleation.
  D. Moth-eaten fibers.
  E. Target fibers.
  F. Ragged red fibers.
  G. Central cores.
  H. Ring fibers.
  I. Aggregates.

NOTE: System for reviewing a muscle biopsy should include evaluation of the supporting tissues, paying particular attention to blood vessels, nerve, connective tissue, muscle spindles and any infiltrates present. Examination of the muscle fiber itself should pay special regard to the presence of:

A. Small angular fibers (Fig 10–3).
B. Change in fiber morphology including size, number, and distribution.
C. Cell nuclei (number and location) (Fig 10–4).
D. Degenerative/regenerative changes.
E. Cellular response (Fig 10–5).
F. Architectural alterations.

All of these changes are best evaluated on transverse sections, although longitudinal sections are valuable for finding nuclear chains and extensive degenerative changes.

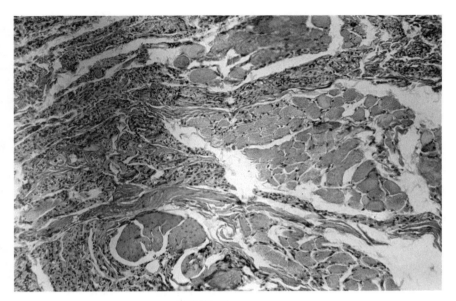

FIG 10–3.
Neuropathic atrophy.

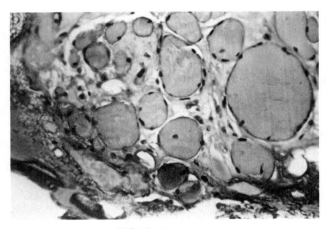

FIG 10–4.
Myopathic atrophy.

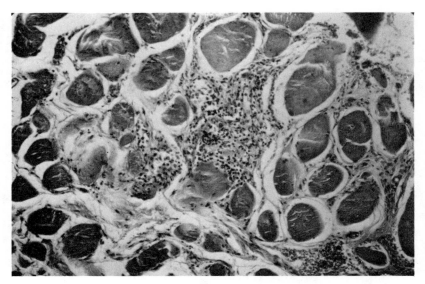

FIG 10–5.
Polymyositis.

NOTE: Certain congenital (morphologically specific) myopathies may be diagnosed by light microscopy (central core disease, nemaline [rod body] myopathy,* myotubular [central nuclear] myopathy). Those requiring electron microscopy for diagnosis include multicore disease, sarcotubular myopathy, finger print myopathy, mitochondrial myopathy, and myopathy with tubular aggregates.

NERVE BIOPSY

This technique is valuable in the diagnosis of diseases of peripheral nerve. Usually the sural (sensory) nerve is the preferred site. With proper histological technique, one can distinguish (1) axonal (Wallerian) degeneration and (2) segmental demyelination (as well as remyelination with onion bulb formation).

The classical histopathological findings in the neuropathies, myopathies, and polymyositis are outlined in Table 10–1.

---

*Rods can be seen after tenotomy, in rhabdomyosarcomas, in some cases of dermatomyositis, and sometimes at the neuromuscular junction in otherwise normal biopsies.

TABLE 10–1.
Comparison of Major Histologic Findings During Active Phase of Common Neuromuscular Disorders*

Neuropathy

Grouped atrophic fibers (sometimes scattered) that are angular (sometimes rounded) on cross-section, and often stained darker than normal, with ATPase and NADH reactions. The electrical counterpart of such type grouping is the giant motor potential.

Modest increase in endomysial connective tissue (less than in myopathy).

Internal nuclei occurring in middle or later stages of the disease.

Pyknotic nuclear clumps.

Bundles of atrophic small fibers interspersed with bundles of normal-sized, normally innervated fibers.

"Targetoid" fibers.

Myopathy

Phagocytosis and necrosis of muscle fibers, preceded by swelling and loss of cross-striations.

Scattered degenerating/regenerating fibers (can occur as a minor feature in neuropathy).

Marked increase of endomysial connective tissue, with deposition of fat.

Hyaline, granular, and fatty degeneration.

Increased number of nuclei and nuclear migration to center of muscle fibers in the early, mid-, or later stages of the disease.

Enlarged nuclei enclosing large nucleoli.

Admixture of small (myogenously deinnervated), normal, and large fibers, all rounded on cross-section.

In early DMD, necrotic or regenerating fibers are found in small, homogeneous groups. However, on the whole, the entire skeletal muscle is involved, with subtle or advanced architectural alteration, with no interspersing of bundles of normal fibers.†

Inflammatory myopathy

Aggregates of inflammatory cells (also can be seen in the early stages of DMD).

Segmental necrosis.

Fiber degeneration/regeneration.

Interstitial edema and/or fibrosis.

Phagocytosis of necrotic fibers.

Perivasculitis.

Perifascicular muscle fiber atrophy.

---

*So-called "myopathic" features may occur in states of chronic denervation. Denervation may accompany many primary myopathies (e.g., polymyositis).
†End-stage neuropathy is difficult to distinguish from end-stage myopathy. In both instances, there is increase of areolar tissue, with profound muscle degeneration and loss of normal architecture.

BIBLIOGRAPHY

Banker BQ (ed): Research in muscle development and the muscle spindle. Exerpta Medica Foundation 1972.

Carpenter S, Karpati G: *Pathology of Skeletal Muscle*. New York, Churchill Livingstone, Inc, 1984.

Dubowitz V, Brooke MH: *Muscle Biopsy: A Modern Approach*. Philadelphia, WB Saunders Co, 1973.

Engel WK: Investigative approach to the muscular dystrophies, in Griggs R, Moxley R, III (eds): *Advances in Neurology*, vol 17. New York, Raven Press, 1977, pp 197–225.

Greenfield JG, Shy GM, Alvord EC, Jr, et al: *An Atlas of Muscle Pathology in Neuromuscular Diseases*. New York, Churchill Livingstone, Inc, 1957.

Jackson MJ, Jones DA, Edward RHT: Vitamin E and muscle diseases. *J Inher Metabol Dis* 1985; 8:84–87.

Milhorat AT (ed): Exploratory concepts in muscular dystrophy and related disorders. Excerpta Medica Foundation 1967.

Sarnat HB: *Muscle Pathology and Histochemistry*. Chicago, American Society of Clinical Pathologists Press, 1983.

11

Genetics

"Alas, our frailty is the cause, not we! For such as we are made of, such we be."

William Shakespeare (1564–1616),*Twelfth Night* II, 2, 32.

Most neuromuscular diseases are genetically determined, consanguinity increasing the risk of occurrence. As a general rule, dominant traits are less severe than recessive ones and gene expression in autosomal-dominant disorders is highly variable. Lethal dominant traits disappear and dominant nonlethal genes tend to be structural abnormalities or changes in nonenzyme proteins, whereas recessively inherited traits lean toward inborn metabolic errors or enzyme defects. The hereditary patterns for the most common types of muscle disease are as follows (Fig 11–1, Tables 11–1, 11–2):

CARRIER STATE

In Duchenne muscular dystrophy (as well as any other X-linked disease), it is important to counsel mothers and female siblings of patients concerning risk of pregnancy.* Bayesian statistical tables are available

---

*Approximately 15% of all Duchenne dystrophics are born as "secondary" cases (where parents are unaware of the presence of the disease in an older child). The mean age at diagnosis of DMD has been reported as ranging from 4.5 to 5.5 years.

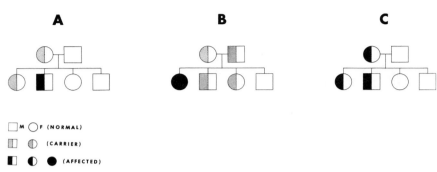

FIG 11–1.
Patterns of genetic determination for the most common types of muscular dystrophy. **A,** X-linked heredity (classic Duchenne dystrophy), carried only by females and transmitted only to males; 50% risk of each male child having the disease and 50% risk of each female being born a carrier. Were a male with X-linked dystrophy to procreate, none of his sons could have the disease, and all of his daughters would be carriers, unless his mate were a carrier, in which case each son and daughter would stand a 50% risk of inheriting the disease. **B,** autosomal recessive heredity (limb girdle dystrophy). Both parents carry the defective gene. There is a 25% risk (regardless of sex) of transmitting the disease, and a 50% risk (regardless of sex) of transmitting the carrier state. **C,** autosomal dominant heredity (facioscapulohumeral dystrophy). Either parent has the disease; there is no carrier state. There is a 50% risk for any child (regardless of sex) inheriting the disease.

for calculation of the jeopardy for a mother or sister with, respectively, an affected son or brother. Risk is based on the number of normal males in the family and the CPK of the concerned female as well as that of her mother (Fig 11–2). As a suspected carrier mother has normal male children, her chances of having a son with the disease are less (Table 11–3). The Bayesian formula (utilizing independent variables to calculate aggregate risk) for computing this risk is $1/2N + 1$ (where N = number of normal births). The risk of a daughter whose CPK is normal, whose mother's CPK is normal and whose brother has DMD, is only 1:52 that she will give birth to a dystrophic son. If, however, her mother has an elevated CPK (even though her own CPK is normal), the hazard rises to 1:16. The chance of a sporadic occurrence of DMD is 1:4,000. If the maternal grandfather is over 35 years of age at the time of the mother's birth, there is an increased chance of that mother being a carrier. Where a single affected male represents a sporadic neomutation, there is a 1:3 gamble that the mother is normal and will not have another male child with muscular dystrophy. The mutation rate for a potentially lethal X-linked condition in which the fertility of affected males is practically zero is one-third. Estimates based on

TABLE 11–1.
Genetic Risks for Most Common Types of Muscular Dystrophy

TYPE	GENETIC PATTERN	AFFECTED RISK	CARRIER RISK	MISCELLANEOUS
Duchenne	Sex-Linked Recessive	Each Male 50%	Each Female 50%	One-third or more of all cases due to sporadic mutation
Limb-girdle	Autosomal Recessive	Each Child 25%	Each Child 50%	Affected rise 100% if both parents exhibit clinical disease
Facioscapulohumeral	Autosomal Dominant	Each Child 50%	0	Fully penetrant trait
Dystrophia myotonica*	Autosomal Dominant	Each Child 50%	0	Variable expressivity. Formes fruste occur

*If the mother has the disease, it usually presents in an affected child at birth. If the father has the disease, it usually presents in an affected child in adolescence or young adulthood.

TABLE 11–2.
Heritability of Selected Neuromuscular Diseases (1981)*

DISEASE	AUTOSOMAL DOMINANT	AUTOSOMAL RECESSIVE	X-LINKED
MUSCULAR DYSTROPHIES			
Duchenne muscular dystrophy	-	1+	4+
Becker muscular dystrophy	-	-	4+
Facioscapulo-humeral	4+	-	-
Limb-girdle	-	4+	-
Myotonic dystrophy	4+	1+	-
Congenital	1+	2+	1+
Ophthalmoplegic	4+	-	-
Distal	2+	-	-
Late onset	2+	-	-
SPINAL MUSCULAR ATROPHIES			
Amyotrophic lateral sclerosis	2+	-	-
Juvenile	-	4+	-
Werdnig-Hoffmann disease	-	4+	-
Kugelberg-Welander disease	2+	2+	-
Benign congenital hypotonia	-	2+	-
Adult progressive			
Proximal	-	2+	-
Distal	2+	-	-
MYOTONIAS			
Myotonia congenita	4+	2+	-
Paramyotonia	4+	-	-

METABOLIC DISEASES OF MUSCLE			
Glycogen storage	-	4+	-
Carnitine deficiency	-	4+	-
Carnitine palmityl transferase	-	4+	-
Periodic paralysis	2+	2+	2+
Endocrinopathies		Very little information	
Malignant hyperthermia	4+	-	-
INFLAMMATORY MYOPATHIES			
Polymyositis		No information	
Dermatomyositis		No information	
DISEASES OF PERIPHERAL NERVE			
Charcot-Marie-Tooth	4+	4+	4+
Friedreich ataxia	1+	4+	-
DISEASES OF NEUROMUSCULAR JUNCTION			
Myasthenia gravis	2+	1+	-
LESS COMMON MYOPATHIES			
Central core disease	4+	-	-
Nemaline myopathy	2+	-	-
Mitochondrial	2+	3+	-
Myotubular myopathy	-	4+	4+

*Courtesy of Elsas LJ, II, Professor of Pediatrics, Director, Division of Medical Genetics, Emory University, Atlanta, Georgia. Used by permission.
1+ –4+ denotes subjective evidence supporting pattern of mendelian inheritance.

TABLE 11–3.
Bayesian Risk Table*

C.P.K.†	CONSULTAND	CONSULTAND'S MOTHER	NORMAL SONS (N2)				NORMAL BROTHERS (N1)								
			0	1	2	3	0	1	2	3	4	5	6	7	8
	+		+				0.3333	0.2500	0.1667	0.1000	0.0556	0.0294	0.0152	0.0077	0.0039
				+			0.2000	0.1429	0.0909	0.0526	0.0286	0.0149	0.0076	0.0039	0.0019
					+		0.1111	0.0769	0.0476	0.0270	0.0145	0.0075	0.0038	0.0019	0.0010
						+	0.0588	0.0400	0.0244	0.0137	0.0073	0.0038	0.0019	0.0010	0.0005
	N		+				0.1493	0.1047	0.0656	0.0375	0.0202	0.0105	0.0054	0.0027	0.0014
				+			0.0806	0.0552	0.0339	0.0191	0.0102	0.0053	0.0027	0.0014	0.0007
					+		0.0420	0.0284	0.0172	0.0097	0.0051	0.0027	0.0013	0.0007	0.0003
						+	0.0215	0.0144	0.0087	0.0048	0.0026	0.0013	0.0007	0.0003	0.0002
	N	N	+				0.0835	0.0498	0.0275	0.0145	0.0075	0.0038	0.0019	0.0018	0.0005
				+			0.0436	0.0255	0.0140	0.0073	0.0038	0.0019	0.0018	0.0005	0.0002
					+		0.0223	0.0129	0.0070	0.0037	0.0019	0.0018	0.0005	0.0002	0.0001
						+	0.0113	0.0065	0.0035	0.0018	0.0009	0.0005	0.0002	0.0001	0.1001
			+				0.6667	0.6000	0.5556	0.5294	0.5152	0.5077	0.5039	0.5019	0.5010
				+			0.5000	0.4286	0.3846	0.3600	0.3469	0.3402	0.3368	0.3351	0.3342

0.3333	0.2727	0.2381	0.2195	0.2099	0.2050	0.2029	0.2012	0.2006
0.2000	0.1579	0.1351	0.1233	0.1172	0.1142	0.1127	0.1119	0.1115
0.4124	0.3448	0.3049	0.2830	0.2716	0.2657	0.2627	0.2612	0.2605
0.2597	0.2083	0.1799	0.1648	0.1571	0.1532	0.1512	0.1502	0.1497
0.1493	0.1163	0.0988	0.0898	0.0853	0.0830	0.0818	0.0812	0.0809
0.0806	0.0617	0.0520	0.0470	0.0445	0.0433	0.0426	0.0423	0.0422
0.3216	0.2920	0.2762	0.2681	0.2639	0.2618	0.2608	0.2603	0.2600
0.1916	0.1710	0.1602	0.1548	0.1520	0.1506	0.1499	0.1496	0.1494
0.1059	0.0935	0.0871	0.0839	0.0823	0.0815	0.0811	0.0808	0.0807
0.0559	0.0490	0.0455	0.0438	0.0429	0.0425	0.0422	0.0421	0.0421

*From Emery AEH, et al: *Genetic Counseling in Muscular Dystrophy.* Amsterdam, Excerpta Medica International Congress, Series No 175, 1967. Used by permission.

†Consultand with an affected brother, N1 normal brothers, and N2 normal sons. It is assumed that two-thirds of known carriers have C.P.K. levels greater than the normal 95 percentile (N).

This table demonstrates the chances of a consultand being a carrier of Duchenne muscular dystrophy. The term *consultand* refers to the female seeking genetic advice with either an affected brother or an affected son (both situations are covered in separate sections of the table.). The figures are for suspect females who have normal CPKs. If the CPK is elevated, the individual is by definition a carrier and the table does not apply. In addition to the number of normal brothers and normal sons, the table also considers whether the consultand's mother has a normal CPK level or whether the CPK has not been determined either on herself or her mother (indicated by blank spaces in the appropriate columns). If the consultand's CPK is half the upper level of normal, the probability is decreased by one-half the indicated value. It can be proportionally reduced further depending upon the specific CPK value. Probability statistics are presented as decimals. As an example, if a mother has a single affected son, a normal CPK, three normal sons and two normal brothers, and her mother's CPK is not available, the chances of her being a carrier of Duchenne muscular dystrophy would be .052 (slightly over 5%) and the odds of her having an affected son are one-fourth of this.

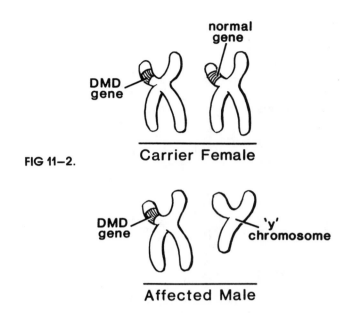

FIG 11–2.   Carrier Female

Affected Male

DMD population studies have produced a similarly high figure. Thus, approximately one-third of mothers of sons with DMD are not carriers, and the disease can be classified as sporadic.

Compliance with recommendations concerning pregnancy in at-risk subjects is variable at best and depends on both the severity of the condition* in question and the statistical risk factor. Genetic counseling should inform more than advise. On the average, each seemingly healthy person carries an abnormal "genetic load" of perhaps four deleterious genes. The chance of genetic abnormality in children born to "normal" parents without familial history of genetic disease lies somewhere between 3% and 8%.

Carriers may be categorized as follows:†

• Definite. Mothers of an affected son who also have an affected brother, maternal uncle, sister's son, or other dystrophic male relatives in the female line of inheritance. A mother may also have affected sons by different, nonsanguineous fathers.

---

*Estimating a consultand's risk is only one aspect of genetic counseling. Equally important is providing information on the burden of the disease; that is, its social, psychological, and medical impact on the patient and his family.

†In calculating risk, it is important to obtain genealogical information on the number of unaffected male relatives and their relationship to the consultand, as well as the results of heterozygote tests in both the female in question and as many of her female relations as possible along the x-chromosomal pathway of the pedigree.

- Probable. Mothers of two or more sons with muscular dystrophy who have no other affected relatives.
- Possible. Mothers of isolated cases, and sisters and other female relatives of affected males.

   Possible carriers may have a known risk (e.g., daughter of a definite carrier [where the risk is 50%] or an unknown risk [sister of a sporadic case]).

DETECTION OF CARRIERS

   I. CPK—increased in approximately 70%–75% of carriers.
      A. A much higher detection rate in childhood. The best time to test for elevated CPK is before age 10 (the age at which it begins to decrease in the average DMD). It is highest in the first few months of life, falls until age 4, increases and peaks by age 10–12, decreasing with the onset of menstruation. It then continues to decline until age 40, when it rises slightly.
      B. Average three samples drawn during different resting states.
      C. Less useful in relatives of patients with any of the less acute, usually autosomal hereditary myopathies.
  II. Serum aldolase, SGOT, SGPT, LDH, and pyruvate kinase can also be elevated in carriers.
 III. Myoglobinemia has been reported in carriers.
  IV. Mild physical findings such as limb-girdle muscle weakness and/or cramping, and calf enlargement (often unilateral). Such symptoms and signs are found in approximately 8% of carriers.
   V. Scattered myopathic EMG changes, particularly quantitative changes.
      A. Determination of absolute refractory period of muscle fibers.
      B. Measurement of the duration and number of phases of motor unit action potentials.
      C. Analysis of the interference pattern by use of an automatic spike counter and computer.
  VI. EKG changes resembling the cardiomyopathy of DMD (without clinical evidence of cardiac disease).
 VII. Slight myopathic changes on biopsy, particularly noted with electron microscopy.
VIII. An increase in in vitro polyribosomal protein synthesis.
  IX. Tissue changes in thigh muscles investigated with ultrasound and CT.
   X. Recombinant DNA linkage studies on extended pedigree.

Duchenne dystrophics seldom survive to reproduce. In benign x-linked (Becker) dystrophy, affected males may survive and have children. All daughters born to such a father will be carriers, and all sons normal (unless, of course, the mother is a carrier, in which case each son and daughter is at 50% risk of inheriting the disease).

Generally speaking, as the genetics become progressively more obscure, so does the prognosis for an individual couple improve because every complication of the simple mendelian scheme lowers the probability of transmitting an abnormal gene.

A fetus can be sexed by amniocentesis at 16–20 weeks of pregnancy, and a therapeutic abortion performed (if desired) if it is a male in a proven carrier. Risks of this procedure include a 1:1,000 rate of infection and a 1:200 incidence of spontaneous abortion. First trimester fetal sexing is possible with chorionic biopsy. This procedure is also useful for linkage studies on the short arm of the X-chromosome at the locus of the DMD gene. Fetal CPK is unreliable as a diagnostic indicator of DMD.

MUSCULAR DYSTROPHY IN YOUNG FEMALES

A young female suffering from what appears to be a disease like Duchenne muscular dystrophy may:

I. Be a manifesting carrier—lyonization (Fig 11–3) (random inactivation in each cell of one X chromosome, which can be either the paternal [normal] or maternal [abnormal] X chromosome) with mosaic abiotrophy.
II. Have benign spinal muscular atrophy of Kugelberg-Welander.
III. Have polymyositis.
IV. Have limb-girdle dystrophy or other autosomal recessive myopathy.
V. Have x-linked disease.
   A. Turner's syndrome (X-O gonadal dysgenesis), XO/XX mosaicism, a structurally abnormal X chromosome, or a translocation with partial deletion of the chromosome.
   B. Result from mating a carrier or normal female who has produced an ovum with a mutant X with a normal male who has produced a sperm carrying a mutant X.*

---

*A female with an affected father and a carrier mother is at 50% risk of inheriting the disease as a homozygote. Needless to say, this is rarely seen.

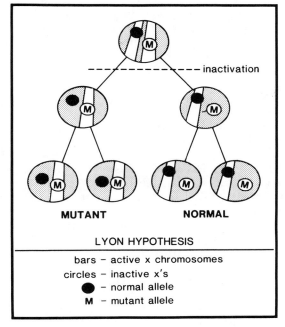

FIG 11–3.

LYON HYPOTHESIS

bars – active x chromosomes
circles – inactive x's
● – normal allele
M – mutant allele

Under ideal conditions of carrier detection, only about two-thirds of those mothers who might give birth to a son with DMD could be discovered. Utilizing therapeutic abortion performed if fetal cells indicate a male chromosomal pattern, allowing only females to come to term, would inevitably lead to the birth of more carriers. Under such circumstances, there is an increased chance of the family forgetting or denying the carrier of muscular dystrophy in its pedigree, and ultimately the population of children with DMD would increase rather than decrease. By far the best course for all known carriers of DMD is to avoid pregnancy and adopt children if they desire a family.

BIBLIOGRAPHY

Adams RD, Denny-Brown D, Pearson CM: *Diseases of Muscle—A Study in Pathology: Hoeber Medical Books.* New York, Harper & Row, 1962.

Bourne GH, Golarz MN (eds): *Muscular Dystrophy in Man and Animals.* Basel, S. Karger, 1963.

Danieli GA, Angeline C: Duchenne carrier detection (letter). *Lancet* 1976; 2:90.

Emery AEH: Genetic counselling in X-linked muscular dystrophy. *J Neurol Sci* 1969; 8:579–587.

Emery AEH: Electrophoretic pattern of lactic dehydrogenase in carriers and patients with Duchenne muscular dystrophy. *Nature* 1964; 201:1044–1045.

Emery AEH: Muscle histology in carriers of Duchenne muscular dystrophy. *J Med Genet* 1965; 2:1–6.

Fowler WM, Gardner GW, Taylor RG, et al: Quantitative measurements in female siblings and mothers of boys with Duchenne dystrophy. *Arch Phys Med Rehab* 1969 50:301–310.

Ionasescu V, Zellweger H: Duchenne muscular dystrophy in young girls. *Acta Neurol Scand* 1974; 50:619–730.

Ionasescu V, Zellweger H, Shirk P, et al: Identification of carriers of Duchenne muscular dystrophy by muscle protein synthesis. *Neurology (Minneapolis)* 1973; 23:497–502.

Mann O, DeLeon AC, Jr, Perloff JK, et al: Duchenne's muscular dystrophy: The electrocardiogram in female relatives. *Am J Med Sci* 1968; 255:376–381.

Moser H: Duchenne muscular dystrophy: Pathogenetic aspects and genetic prevention. *Hum Genet* 1984; 66:17–40.

Moser H, Emery AEH: The manifesting carrier in Duchenne muscular dystrophy. *Clin Genet* 1974; 5:271–284.

Pearn JH: Patients: Subjective interpretation of risks offered in genetic counselling. *J Med Genet* 1973; 10:129–134.

Penn AS, Lisak RP, Rowland LP: Muscular dystrophy in young girls. *Neurology* 1970; 20:147–159.

Roses AD, Roses MJ, Miller SE, et al: Carrier detection in Duchenne muscular dystrophy. *N Engl J Med* 1976; 294:193–198.

Roses MS, Nicholson MT, Kircher CS, et al: Evaluation and detection of Duchenne's and Becker's muscular dystrophy carriers by manual muscle testing. *Neurology* 1977; 27:20–25.

Rott H, Santellani M, Rodl W, et al: Duchenne muscular dystrophy: Carrier detection by ultrasound and computerized tomography. *Lancet* 1983; 19:1199–2000.

Skinner R, Emery AEH: Serum-creatine-kinase levels in carriers of Becker muscular dystrophy. *Lancet* 1974; 2:1023–1024.

Smith I, Thomson WHS: Carrier detection in X-linked (Duchenne) muscular dystrophy: Pyruvate kinase isoenzymes and creatine phosphokinase in serum and blood cells. *Clin Chim Acta* 1977; 78:439–451.

Symposium on Genetics of Congenital Deformity; Clinical Orthopaedics and Related Research, vol 33. Philadelphia, JB Lippincott, Co. 1964.

Wilson KM, Evans KA, Carter CO: Creatine kinase levels in women who carry genes for three types of muscular dystrophy. *Br Med J* 1965; 1:750–753.

12

X-ray

"One look is worth a thousand listens."

Merrill C. Sosman (1890–1959)

All of the roentgen changes in bone seen in the myopathies occur because of muscular weakness, atrophy, and/or contracture. They do not express a primary mesodermal or mineral defect. X-ray features in muscular dystrophy, although not pathognomonic of the disease, include:

I. Osteoporosis. This late change in advanced disease is due to muscular weakness and disuse (Fig 12–1). Epiphyses sometimes show a radiolucent center surrounded by a peripheral, thin, dense line (signet ring appearance) while profound demineralization is noted in the remainder of the bone.

II. Talipes equinocavovarus (Fig 12–2). In the advanced stages of dystrophy, abnormal posture due to unopposed muscle contraction causes this as well as other deformities.

III. Vertebral caninization (Fig 12–3). The relative height of the vertebral bodies (which may ultimately become square in shape) is increased, as in the quadriped. This change is seen in children chronically bedridden for any cause.

IV. Decreased tibial diameter (Fig 12–4). This finding is usually ac-

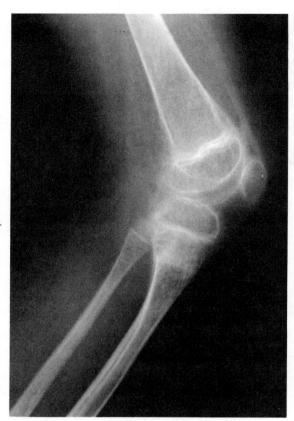

FIG 12–1.
Osteoporosis.

companied by increased a.p. fibular thickness with decreased frontal fibular diaphyseal diameter. It is due to a lack of growth stimulation secondary to normal muscular tension and can be noted after age 6. It is found in the childhood myopathies. The lateral x-ray will often show the width of the middle third of the tibial diaphysis to be no larger than that of its adjacent fibula. Normal lateral fibula/tibia ratio is less than 0.66. In DMD it is above 0.70. Linear (enchondral) growth is not so much affected as circumferential (membranous) growth in the long bones be-cause circumferential growth depends on normal muscular ten-sile function.

V. Overtubulation of long bone shafts (Fig 12–5). Early onset mus-cular dystrophy can result in the long bones becoming thin with

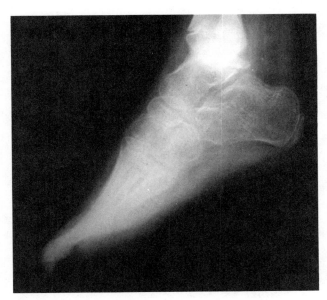

FIG 12–2.
Talipes equinocavovarus.

decrease in their diaphyseal cortex and narrowing of their med-
ullary canals (concentric atrophy).

VI. Symmetric diminution in the size of the scapula is often found
in dystrophies with childhood onset.

VII. Small pelvis with prominent ischial spines and flaring iliac
bones (Fig 12–6). These changes are noted when a child is confined early to a wheelchair.

VIII. Increased soft tissue shadow (in areas of hypertrophy and
"pseudohypertrophy" (Fig 12–7). With hypertrophy, the soft tissue density is that of muscle, but with "pseudohypertrophy," it
becomes striated with shadows of lipid density secondary to
fatty infiltration. This is a late phenomenon. Conversely, decreased soft tissue shadow indicative of muscular atrophy can
be seen in SMA, arthrogryposis, or any other neuromuscular
disease in which atrophy is a feature.

IX. Valgus hip deformity (Fig 12–8) (femoral neck angle often
greater than 140 degrees) This deformity is due to lack of muscle
tension about the hip. Subluxation may ensue.

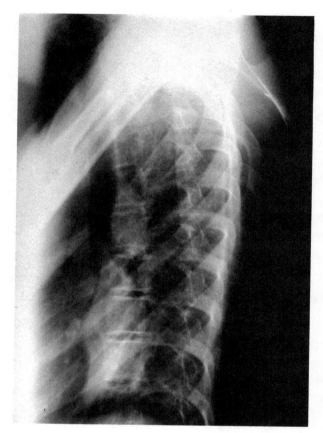

FIG 12–3.
Vertebral caninization.

X. Standing lordosis (early) and scoliosis (late) with occasional ky-
   phosis. See sections on pathomechanics and scoliosis for a full
   explanation of these findings.
XI. Moderate retardation of bone age.
XII. In dermatomyositis:
   A. Obliteration of normal soft tissue planes and swelling caused
      by edema.
   B. Nasogastric reflux (barium) during swallowing.
   C. Reduced peristalsis with dilatation and thickening of the
      small bowel.
   D. Gastric and/or duodenal ulceration.

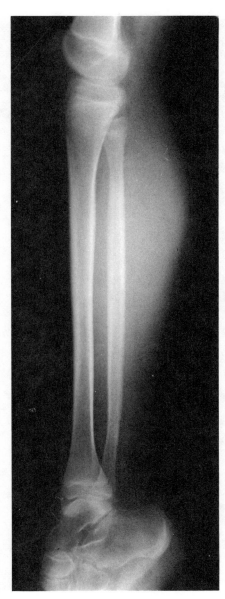

FIG 12–4.
Decreased tibial diameter.

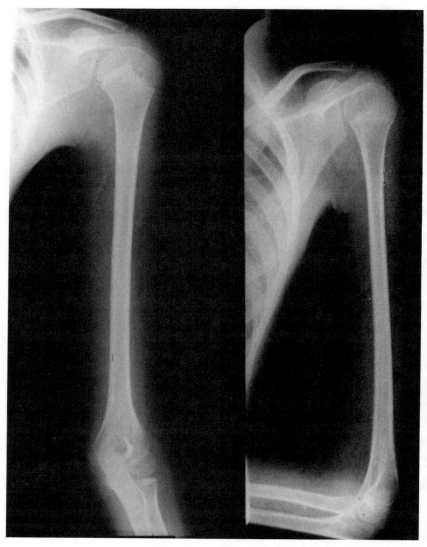

FIG 12–5.
Long bone overtubulation.

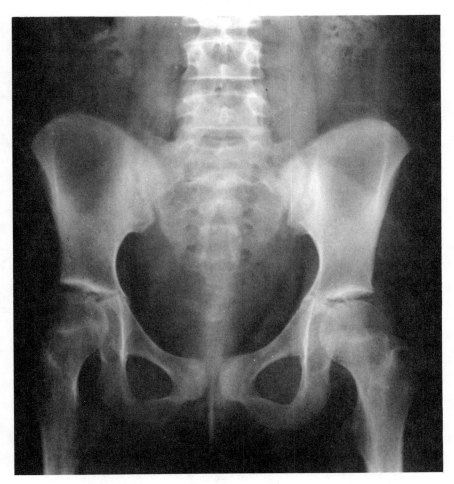

FIG 12–6.
Small pelvis/prominent ischial spines/flaring iliac bones.

     E. Soft tissue calcification secondary to inflammation.
XIII. X-ray findings described in dystrophia myotonica.
     A. Esophageal dysfunction, including inability to swallow a nor-
       mal-sized bolus, poor peristalsis, and barium pooling in the
       pharynx.
     B. Colonic atony on barium enema (secondary to smooth mus-
       cle involvement).
     C. Changes in the skull, including a small sella turcica, hyper-

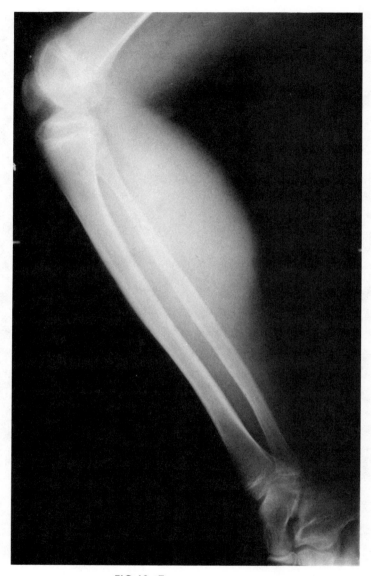

FIG 12–7.
Increased soft tissue shadow.

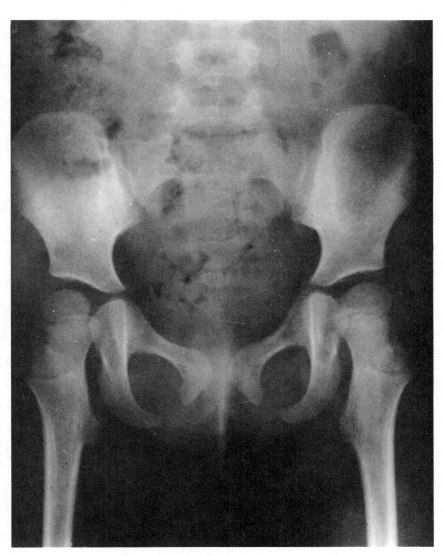

FIG 12–8.
Valgus hip deformity.

ostosis frontalis, liontiasis ossea, large frontal sinuses, and poor mandibular angle.
  D. Elevation of the diaphragm secondary to phrenic nerve atrophy.
  E. Basal atelectasis and pneumonitis (probably from aspiration) can be noted in advanced cases. Cardiomegaly may be recognized roentgenographically.
XIV. The major computerized tomographic findings in myopathy are early diffuse or spotty density changes within muscle. Fascia is unaffected. Atrophy occurs later. In neural diseases, atrophy is seen before decreased muscle density is apparent. Studies with ultrasound have also disclosed changes in muscle texture with disease, as has examination by magnetic resonance imaging.

BIBLIOGRAPHY

Bulcke JAL: Commentary: Ultrasound and CT scanning in the diagnosis of neuromuscular diseases, in Gamstrop I, Sarnat HB (eds): *Progressive Spinal Muscular Atrophies.* New York, Raven Press, 1984, pp 153–161.

Edwards RHT, Griffiths RD, Hayward M, et al: Modern methods of diagnosis of muscle diseases. *J R Coll Physicians Lond* 1986; 20:49–55.

Epstein BS, Abramson JL: Roentgenologic changes in the bones in cases of pseudohypertrophic muscular dystrophy. *Arch Neurol Psychiatry* 1941; 46:868–876.

Gay BB, Jr, Weems HS: Roentgenologic evaluation of disorders of muscle. *Semin Roentgenol* 1973; 8:25.

Hawley RJ, Schellinger D, O'Doherty DS: Computed tomographic patterns of muscles in neuromuscular diseases. *Arch Neurol* 1984; 41:343–387.

Heckmatt JZ, Dubowitz V: Diagnosis of spinal muscular atrophy with pulse echo ultrasound imaging, in Gamstrop I, Sarnat HB (eds): *Progressive Spinal Muscular Atrophies.* New York, Raven Press, 1984, pp 141–151.

Heckmatt JZ, Dubowitz V, Leeman S: Detection of pathological change in dystrophic muscle with B-scan ultrasound imaging. *Lancet* 1980; 1:1389–1390.

Lewitan A, Nathanson L: The Roentgen features of muscular dystrophy. *Am J Roentgenol* 1955; 73:226–234.

O'Doherty DS, Schellinger D, Raptopoulos V: Computed tomographic patterns of pseudohypertrophic muscular dystrophy: Preliminary results. *J Comput Assist Tomogr* 1977; 1:482–486.

PART III

Classification and Diagnosis of Neuromuscular Diseases

13

Classification

"Disease is very old, and nothing about it has changed. It is we who change as we learn to recognize what was formerly imperceptible."
    Jean Marie Charcot (1825–1893), *De L'Expectation en Medecine*
"Disease often tells its secrets in a casual parenthesis."
Wilfred Trotter (1872–1939), Collected papers, *Art and Science in Medicine*

There are numerous neuromuscular diseases. These can be broadly classified into major disease categories of (1) spinal muscular atrophies, (2) peripheral neuropathies, (3) disease of the myoneural junction, and (4) myopathies. Groups 1, 2, and 3 are primary diseases "of" neural tissues (secondarily "in" muscle). Group 4 comprises diseases "of" muscle (Table 13–1). Further subgrouping can be made on (1) genetic basis, where known, (2) clinical course, (3) histopathologic changes, (4) presence of nerve or muscle toxins, (5) characteristic laboratory findings, and (6) association with other medical diseases. A practical classification of those neuromuscular disorders most frequently seen follows.

ANTERIOR HORN CELL DISEASES

Spinal Muscular Atrophies

Due to failure of development or progressive degeneration of the lower motor neuron cell body, with resultant degeneration of the peripheral

TABLE 13–1.
Localization of Neuromuscular Lesions*

CATEGORY	ANTERIOR HORN CELL	PERIPHERAL NERVE	NEUROMUSCULAR JUNCTION	MUSCLE
Creatine phosphokinase	Usually N can be elevated	Normal	Normal	Increased
Electromyography	Fibrillation Polyphasic potentials (group type) Giant potentials Interference pattern reduced	Same as in anterior horn cell	Post exertional decrement of action potentials	Polyphasic potentials (short type) Myotonic discharge Action potential amplitude and duration reduced Normal interference pattern
Nerve conduction	Normal	Reduced	Normal Decrement of evoked potentials during subtetanic stimulation	Normal
Muscle biopsy	Small and large group atrophic fibers Fiber hypertrophy Fiber type grouping Degeneration in cellular response but architectural changes not seen	Same	Selective Type II atrophy (60%) Signs of denervation (25%) Lymphorrhages (35%) (myasthenia gravis)	Degeneration Necrosis Increased connective tissue Internal nuclei

*Modified from Murphy EG, Walsburg H: *Pediatr Clin North Am* 1974; 21:917–926. Used by permission.

motor nerve fibers. Weakness is generally more severe proximally. As cardiomyopathy is rare, prognosis depends on respiratory function.

I. Generally transmitted by an autosomal recessive trait. Affected siblings can show variation in severity and age of onset of the disease. In sibling pairs, the females often outlive the males.

A. Neurogenic findings on physical examination (Fig 13–1): Tongue and eyelid fasciculations, weakness, atrophy, depressed to absent reflexes, seldom contractures, except in the wheelchair patient (postural when they occur), myokymia on muscle percussion, minipolymyoclonus (fine even muscular tremor of all fingers at once, noted in the outstretched hand secondary to

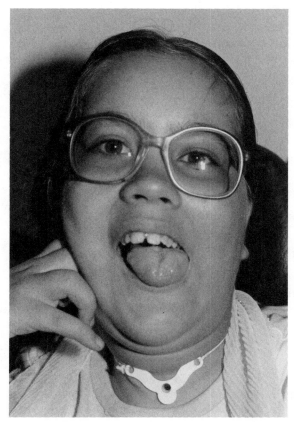

FIG 13–1.
SMA. Note tongue atrophy and tracheostomy.

asynchronous firing of reinnervated muscle fibers), neostig-
mine-induced muscle fasciculations, voluntary contraction fasciculations, contraction fasciculation trembling, palpable contraction fasciculations, and high-intensity, low-pitched rumbling on
skeletal muscle auscultation.
  B. Neuropathic biopsy (large group atrophy with rounded, hypertrophic fibers and some small angular fibers).
  C. EMG. Fibrillation potentials, reduced interference pattern, decreased frequency, increased amplitude, and duration of action
potential.
  D. A higher incidence of seizures than normal.
  E. Variable severity and progression; some cases seem to stabilize
or arrest.
     1. SMA I—acute infantile (Werdnig-Hoffmann disease). Floppy
        newborn: severe disability, unable to sit. Early death due to
        respiratory failure.
     2. SMA II—Intermediate. Able to sit but cannot stand or walk
        unaided. Some survive to adult life. CPK may be slightly in-
        creased.
     3. SMA III—juvenile onset (Kugelberg-Welander disease). Mild
        disability. Able to stand and walk. Most survive to adult life
        with essentially normal life expectancy. CPK may be mod-
        estly increased. EMG can show neurogenic and myopathic
        features. May have myocardial involvement with conduction
        abnormalities.
     4. SMA IV—adult onset of disease with possibly normal life ex-
        pectancy and mild to moderate disability (Table 13–2).

Motor Neuron Disease (Amyotrophic Lateral Sclerosis)

This usually affects adults (40–70 years of age)—men more than
women. It may run a rapid, two years or slower (5–20+ years) course.
Some cases seem to be familial with high incidence among the Cha-
morros of Guam and other Mariana Islands. Others appear to be related to neuronal exhaustion (age, athletics).

  I. Shows both upper and lower motor neuron signs.
 II. Progressive wasting and weakness with fasciculations, hyperre-
     flexia and extensor plantar responses. Must rule out cervical
     spondylotic myelopathy. Also, multiple myeloma, macroglobuli-
     nemia, and neoplasia may each be complicated by anterior horn
     cell disease.

TABLE 13–2.
Adult Onset Conditions That Present With the Clinical Picture of Spinal Muscular Atrophy*

Spinal muscular atrophy
    Adult, sporadic, idiopathic, or familial
    ALS?
Cervical spondylosis
Amyotrophy
    Historically remote poliomyelitis
    Diabetic
    Syphilitic spinal meningitis
    Syringomyelia
    Spinal cord tumors
Late onset peroneal muscular atrophy
Creutzfeldt-Jakob's disease
Shy-Drager syndrome
Multiple sclerosis (rarely)
Familial spinal muscular atrophy, accompanied by Type II
    hyperlipoproteinemia
Spinal muscular atrophy with macroglobulinemia or
    multiple myeloma

*Modified from Richter PL, McMasters RE: *South Med J* 1972; 65:317–320. Used by permission.

III. Bulbar involvement with dysphagia and dysarthria.
    A. Prognosis depends on extent of bulbar involvement.
IV. Sensory symptoms may occur.
 V. Treatment (symptomatic and supportive).
    A. Antispasmodic drugs (e.g., baclofen).
    B. Anticholinergic agents (e.g., atropine).
    C. PT, orthotics, OT aids.
    D. Feeding gastrostomies.
    E. Respiratory support—tracheostomy.

Poliomyelitis

Mild to severe motor loss with variable recovery. It is characterized by febrile illness, GI symptoms, muscle pain and meningeal involvement.

NEUROPATHIES

 I. Genetically determined polyneuropathies (hereditary motor and sensory neuropathy—HMSN) present with a centrifugal pattern of muscle wasting, decreased position, and vibration sense. In the dominantly inherited condition, minor expression of the gene may be encountered in females. They tend to be less severely affected than males. These diseases represent a continuum from Charcot-Marie-Tooth disease through Friedreich's ataxia. Co-occurrence of HMSN and spinocerebellar ataxia in the same family has been reported.

A. HMSN Type I ("hypertrophic" Charcot-Marie-Tooth disease). Peroneal muscular atrophy secondary to demyelinization. Below knee wasting (jambe de coq). Sometimes lower thigh atrophy (inverted champagne bottle thighs).
   1. Onset usually in first decade; genetically heterogenous.
   2. Reflexes lost; muscle spindles show pathology (fibrosis).
   3. May have sensory loss and weakness in both hands and feet (median and ulnar nerves affected in hands) (Fig 13–2).
   4. Nerves enlarged.
      a) Most apparent in peroneal, ulnar, and posterior auricular nerves. Myelographic filling defects at lumbar roots secondary to localized enlargement may mimic filling defect of herniated disc.
      b) Both sensory and motor nerve conduction slow.

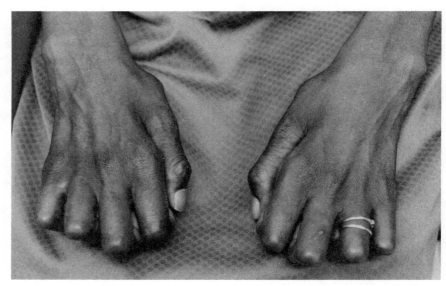

FIG 13–2.
Combined median-ulnar neuropathy in HMSN-1.

      c) Nerve biopsy reveals segmental demyelination and "onion bulbs."

      d) Foot deformity is equinocavovarus with "hammertoes" (Fig 13–3)

      e) Surgery for hand deformity (e.g., opponens plasty) indicated in older patients.

      f) Can be associated with fine tremor of the hands (Roussy-Levy syndrome).

B. HMSN Type II ("neuronal" Charcot-Marie-Tooth disease). Peroneal muscular atrophy secondary to axonal degeneration.

  1. Onset usually in third or fourth decades.

  2. Variable distal sensory signs and weakness in the hands (more commonly and severely present in the feet).

  3. No nerve enlargement.

  4. Sensory nerve conduction may be normal or only slightly slowed, and motor nerve conduction slightly slowed, but decreased amplitude on EMG.

  5. Nerve biopsy shows axonal degeneration.

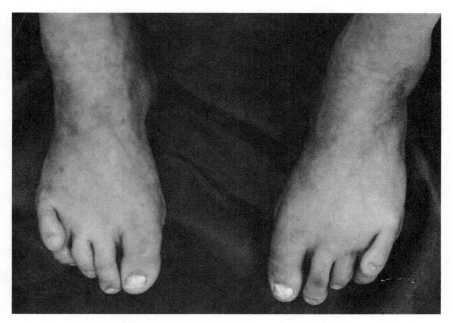

FIG 13–3.
Equinocavovarus with hammertoes in HMSN-1.

    6. Foot deformity is calcaneocavus with "hammertoes" and "stork legs."
       a) Acetabular dysplasia may be present.
       b) Patients at risk for neuropathic ankle arthritis.

C. HMSN Type III (Dejerine-Sottas disease).
    1. Hypertrophic neuropathy of infancy.
    2. CSF protein elevated.
    3. Nerve conduction markedly slowed.
    4. Cavus deformity of feet.
    5. Scoliosis that requires fusion.
    6. Wheelchair confined by third or fourth decade.

D. HMSN Type IV (Refsum's disease).
    1. Hypertrophic neuropathy with excess phytanic acid.
    2. Mimics Friedreich's ataxia.
       a) Onset in first and second decade.
       b) Decreased sensory nerve conduction.
       c) Positive Romberg sign with ataxia.
       d) Cavus foot deformity.
       e) Over 80% have scoliosis.
       f) Usual course leads to wheelchair confinement in late teens or 20s and death from cardiopathy and inanition by the fifth decade.
       g) Nystagmus.
       h) May have remissions/relapses.

E. HMSN Type V (peripheral neuropathy with spastic paraplegia) Friedreich's ataxia (spino-cerebellar degeneration).
    1. Autosomal recessive.
    2. Onset in first or second decade.*
    3. Progressive cerebellar ataxia, impaired lower extremity position sense, cardiomyopathy, kyphoscoliosis, nystagmus.
    4. Initial symptoms usually in the legs (spasticity) with absent reflexes and extensor plantar responses. Later, ataxia of arms and affected speech are noted.† The following associated defects have been reported:
       a) Primary optic atrophy.
       b) Retinitis pigmentosa.
       c) Choroidal sclerosis.

---

  *Spinocerebellar degenerations usually begin in adolescence and follow a subacute course. Cerebellar (or olivopontocerebellar) degenerative disease may manifest in middle or late adulthood, and run a slowly progressive, chronic course.

  †Loss of deep tendon reflexes is due to involvement of dorsal root; dysarthria to cerebellar disease; Babinski signs may be present if corticospinal tract is involved.

d) Cataract.

e) Ptosis.

f) External ocular palsy.

g) Abnormal pupillary reflexes.

h) Deafness.

i) Deaf-mutism.

j) Degeneration of brain-stem motor nuclei.

k) Syndactyly.

l) Polydactyly.

m) Epilepsy.

n) Mental deficiency.

o) Progressive dementia.

p) Diabetes mellitus (25%).

q) Cryptorchidism.

r) Hypogenitalism and obesity.

s) Habitual hyperthermia.

5. Foot deformity secondary to muscle imbalance (preponderance of posterior tibial).

   a) Pes equinus or equinovarus.

   b) Pes cavus.

   c) Claw toes.

   d) Intrinsic muscle wasting.

6. Motor nerve conduction normal. Sensory nerve action potentials reduced or absent. Mild neurogenic changes on EMG of distal muscles.

7. Pathology is in posterior and lateral columns of spinal cord. Nerve biopsy shows axonal degeneration.

8. Management—supportive and symptomatic.

   a) Orthosis.

   b) Foot and spinal corrective surgery.

      Most patients are wheelchair confined by the third decade and many die before age 40 from cardiac complications.

NOTE: Other genetically determined polyneuropathies include metachromatic leukodystrophy, acute intermittent porphyria, and amyloid neuropathy.

II. Acquired neuropathies.

   A. The secondary mononeuropathies can be classed as traumatic, including entrapment and inflammatory.

   B. The acquired polyneuropathies include

      1. Inflammatory; polyradiculoneuropathy (Guillain-Barré syndrome).

2. Neuropathies associated with metabolic diseases such as diabetes mellitus, vitamin deficiencies or alcoholic neuropathy, renal and hepatic disease.
3. Neuropathies due to drugs or toxic agents.
4. Neuropathies seen with malignant disease or infection.
5. Neuropathies accompanying connective tissue disorders.

DISEASES OF THE MYONEURAL JUNCTION

Myasthenia Gravis

This disorder of neuromuscular transmission is due to a reduction of available acetylcholine receptors at neuromuscular junctions (Fig 13–4), brought about by an autoimmune episode and characterized by fluctuating weakness and fatigability; it improves with rest. This fatigability distinguishes myasthenia from the other myopathies.

I. Types.
  A. Neonatal. Occurs in approximately 15% of newborn children of myasthenic mothers, secondary to passive transfer of myasthenic IgG from mother, and is transient although it may be severe and life threatening during the first two weeks after birth.
  B. Congenital. Occasionally evident at birth with dysphagia, respiratory distress, and generalized weakness. More commonly

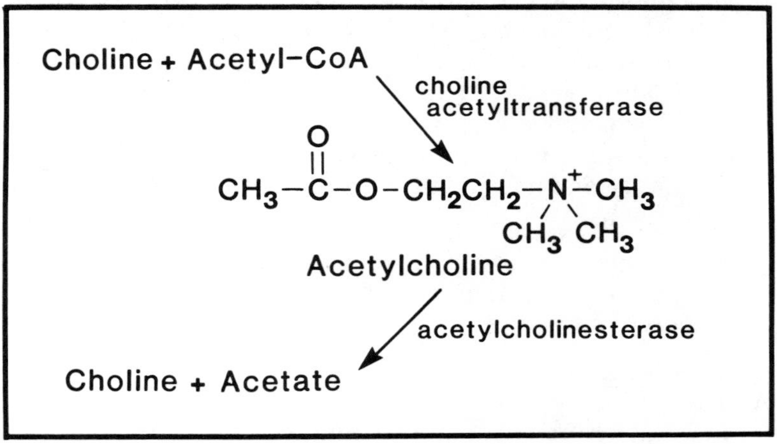

FIG 13–4.
Acetylcholine biosynthesis and catabolism.

present during first two years of life with ptosis or ophthalmoplegia.

C. Juvenile. Resembles adult disease.

D. Adult myasthenia.

E. Drug-induced myasthenia (d-penicillamine).

II. Signs and symptoms.

A. Disease more frequent in females. It is said to be a disease of
older men and younger women (male peak age 60; female
peak age 30). Weakness may be confined to extraocular muscles or generalized (mild, moderate, or severe).

B. Ocular muscles (ptosis) (Fig 13–5), proximal limb muscles (pelvic and pectoral girdles), and bulbar muscles are most commonly involved.

1. Tendon reflexes decreased.

C. Symptoms exacerbated by stress, heat, or repetitive tasks.
Also worsened with infection, menstruation, and pregnancy.

D. Weakness fluctuates, symptoms more evident in PM.

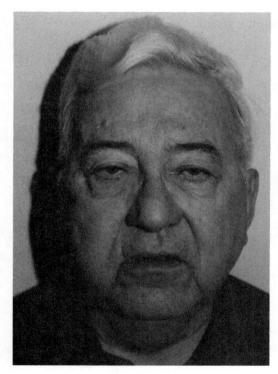

FIG 13–5.
Myasthenia gravis. Note ptosis.

E. Facial muscles can be involved.
F. Spontaneous remissions (25%) and relapses common.
G. Bulbar involvement may lead to voice changes and respiratory difficulty.
H. Neck muscles (particularly extensors) commonly weak.
I. Increased incidence of diabetes, lupus, rheumatoid arthritis, thyrotoxicosis, and cancer. Family history of autoimmune conditions—tuberculosis, ulcers and hypertension.
J. Laboratory workup.
   1. Lupus preps.
   2. Antinuclear antibodies.
   3. Rheumatoid factor.
   4. Antithyroglobulin antibodies.
   5. Thyroid function tests (approximately 5% have thyrotoxicosis).
   6. Pulmonary function tests.
   7. Chest x-ray.
   8. Fasting blood sugar.
   9. Tuberculin test.
   10. CT scan of mediastinum (for thymic tumor or hyperplasia).
III. Pathology.
   A. Myasthenia gravis is a genetic autoimmune disease.
      1. Familial occurrence has been reported in some cases.
   B. The neuromuscular transmission defect is postsynaptic.
   C. The circulating antibody to ACh receptor has been identified in the blood of about 90% of myasthenic patients.
   D. Thymomas occur in approximately 10% of myasthenics, thymic hyperplasia in 70%.
      1. Young females with thymic hyperplasia have high prevalence of HLA-8 antibody (which is uncommon in older males and patients with thymomas).
   E. Lymphorrhages can be found on muscle biopsy.
IV. Diagnosis.
   A. Improvement with test of IM or oral neostigmine or IV edrophonium (Tensilon).
      1. Careful about placebo reactors.
      2. Cover muscarinic effects with atropine.
      3. Can increase weakness with small dose of curare. May require assisted ventilation. Regional curare test safer.
   B. Decremental response of evoked muscle action potential on supramaximal nerve stimulation (this is the electrical counterpart to fatigue on repeated muscle contraction).

1. EMG usually normal but increased neuromuscular jitter on single-fiber EMG.

C. Increase in ACh receptor antibody level.

V. Management.*

A. Anticholinesterase drugs. Adjust dosage empirically to obtain optimal effect. Can use sustained release preparations at night (Table 13–3).

NOTE: Monitor for cholinergic crisis.

B. Thymectomy. For thymoma or if symptoms uncontrolled with anticholinesterase drugs (in patients over 50 years of age). Should wait 6–12 months after onset to exclude early spontaneous remission.

C. Immunosuppressive therapy.

1. Steroids. In a patient uncontrolled by anticholinesterase drugs who is older than 50 years, post-thymectomy or purely ocular myasthenia.

   a) Titrate daily dose gradually to optimal response (usually 50–60 mg prednisone/day).

   b) Slowly switch to alternate-day dosage.

   c) Maintain until improvement plateau reached.

   d) Titrate slowly down to minimal maintenance dose.

   e) Observe precautions for side effects.

2. Azathioprine or 6-mercaptopurine reserved for patients

TABLE 13–3.
Anticholinesterase Drugs Commonly Used for Myasthenia Gravis*

DRUG	ROUTE	ADULT DOSE	CHILD'S DOSE†	NEONATAL AND INFANT DOSE	FREQUENCY
Neostigmine bromide (Prostigmine)	PO	15 mg	10 mg	1–2 mg	q2–3 h
Neostigmine methyl sulfate (Prostigmine injectable)	IM, IV	0.5 mg‡	0.1 mg†	0.05 mg	q2–3 h
Pyridostigmine bromide§ (Mestinon)	PO	60 mg	30 mg	4–10 mg	q3–4 h
	IM, IV	2 mg‡	0.5–1.5 mg/kg	0.1–0.5 mg	q3–4 h
Mestinon/Timespan	PO	180 mg			q8–10 h

*From Walshe TM, III: Diseases of nerve and muscle, in Samuels MA (ed): *Manual of Neurologic Therapeutics*, ed 2. Boston, Little, Brown & Co, 1982. Used by permission.
†The dose in children varies so much that it must be determined for each case. Small amounts of the drug are given and increased as indicated by the clinical improvement.
‡The parenteral dose is usually one-thirtieth of the oral dose.
§Also available as a liquid and as chloride.

*The pharmacologic approach to treating myasthenia gravis is to either enhance neuromuscular transmission or suppress the immune basis of the disease.

unresponsive to steroids or thymectomy. Long-term treatment complicated by bone marrow depression, decreased resistance to infection and neoplasia.
   3. Plasmapheresis. Useful in severe myasthenic crisis.
  D. Avoid:
    1. Curare and other nondepolarizing muscle relaxants.
    2. Sedatives, hypnotics, narcotics, barbiturates, and tranquilizers.
    3. Quinine, procainamide, lidocaine.
    4. Neuromuscular blocking antibiotics.
     a) Streptomycin.
     b) Neomycin.
     c) Gentamicin.

NOTE: Myasthenic syndrome (Eaton-Lambert) associated with malignant tumors (particularly oat-cell carcinoma of the lung) and characterized by proximal muscle weakness (improved with exercise) and decreased deep tendon reflexes. Extraocular muscle weakness and ptosis are rare. There is a male predominance. An *incremental* response to high-frequency repetitive nerve stimulation is noted. The syndrome is due to inadequate release of normal acetylcholine quanta and may be improved with guanidine (administered through a nasogastric tube as it can cause stomal ulceration).

MYOPATHIES

  I. Genetically determined muscular dystrophy.*
   A. Duchenne muscular dystrophy.†
    1. Prevalence is 3 per 100,000 of total population. Occurrence is 1 per 5,000 live male births.
    2. X-linked (30% sporadic, spontaneous mutation rate is estimated at 10^{-5}); disease found in males and carried only by females.
    3. Pregnancy and birth usually normal.
     a) Occasionally mothers relate that child was not very active in utero.
    4. Weakness is symmetrical. Abiotrophy with subsequent

---

*Neither cause nor cure of these conditions is known. Specifically, in spite of hundreds of drug trials, no pharmacologic agent has yet been found that effectively arrests the basic process(es) of these diseases.

†Duchenne muscular dystrophy is the most common X-linked human lethal disease.

atrophy and weakness of striated musculature is found.

  a) Although all skeletal muscle is eventually involved (Fig
     13–6,A), the para-axial and appendicular postural mus-
     cles (of shoulder and pelvic girdles)—those muscles
     first formed in embryo—are involved earliest and most
     severely (Fig 13–6,B). Facial and extraocular muscles re-
     main clinically intact, although macroglossia and hyper-
     trophy of the masseter muscles can be seen.
5. Motor milestones usually somewhat delayed.
  a) Fifty percent fail to walk until 18 months.
6. Early signs include:
  a) Flat feet (secondary to heel-cord contracture).

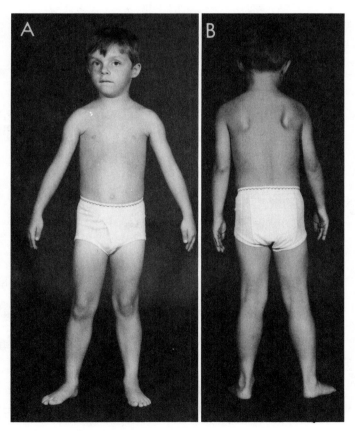

FIG 13–6.
DMD. **A,** frontal view. **B,** posterior view.

   b) Weak shoulder extension.
   c) Hesitance when ascending stairs.
   d) Slight lateral pelvic shift and elevation of buttocks when arising from seated position on floor.
   e) Acceleration during final stage of sitting down.
   f) Poor standing jump.
   g) Waddling run.
 7. Later signs include:
   a) Waddling gait.
   b) Frequent falling.
   c) Difficulty ascending stairs.
   d) Slipping through.
   e) Positive Gowers' (tripod) sign.
   f) Lordosis (Fig 13–7).
   g) Progressive equinus steppage.
   h) Weak neck flexion.
 8. Exercise cramping may occur.
 9. Deep tendon reflexes are depressed as muscles weaken. They tend to cease on the dominant side first. The non-dominant Achilles reflex is usually the last to disappear. This is because the heel cord is the strongest tendon in the body and it tracks a very straight course from origin to insertion. Thus, its muscle spindles are situated in an environment propitious for continued function.
10. True muscle hypertrophy and later pseudohypertrophy (substitution of fat and areolar tissue for muscle) seen in calves (Fig 13–8) (occasionally in deltoids, triceps, serratus anterior, and vastus lateralis muscles) (Fig 13–9).
   a) Enlargement is dependent upon an intact nerve supply.
   b) Involved muscles have a doughy (rubbery) consistency on palpation. The specific gravity of this muscle is less than normal because of replacement by adipose and fibrous tissue.
   c) Masseter and tongue hypertrophy (Fig 13–10,A and B) can occur.
11. Sensation unaffected.
12. Weakness accentuated by immobilization. Loss of ambulation between 9–12 years of age. Death (pulmonary or cardiac) in late teens.
13. Significant number of patients are intellectually impaired.

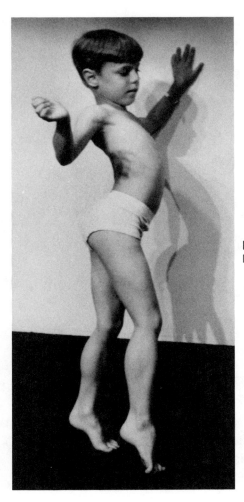

FIG 13–7.
DMD. Lordosis and equinus.

14. Laboratory diagnosis:
    a) Typical EMG.
    b) Typical biopsy.
    c) Markedly increased CPK (at least 10 times normal in early stages, though lower later); increased urinary excretion of 3-methylhistadine.
15. Cardiomyopathy common.
16. Spurious improvement due to normal growth and increase in motor ability at age 5 to 8 years.

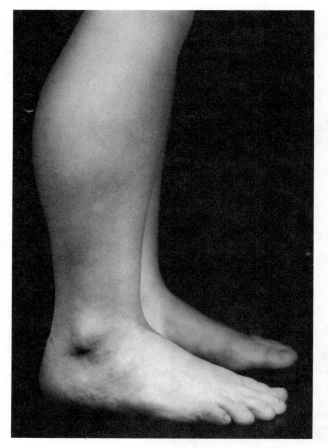

FIG 13—8.
Calf hypertrophy.

    17. No dysphagia or sphincter difficulty.
B. Becker-type dystrophy.
    1. X-linked. This variant constitutes 10% of DMD.
    2. Similar proximal distribution of muscle weakness as in
        Duchenne muscular dystrophy but asymmetrical; usually
        maintains neck flexor strength. May present with pes
        cavus, unusual hypertrophy (thenar eminence), or patellar
        subluxation secondary to quadriceps weakness.
    3. Later onset and patients are ambulatory into third decade
        with longer life expectancy than DMD.

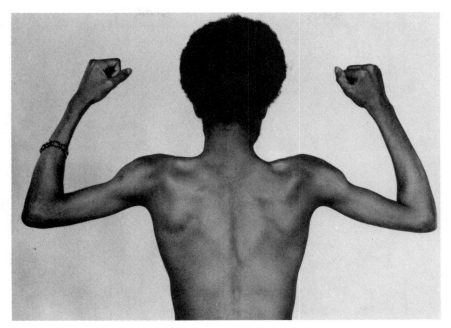

FIG 13–9.
Deltoid hypertrophy.

    a) Triceps power often greater than biceps.
    b) May develop ambulatory scoliosis because of asymmetrical paraspinal muscle weakness.
  4. Laboratory diagnosis:
    a) Increased CPK.
    b) Mixed pattern on EMG.
    c) Biopsy somewhat different than Duchenne dystrophy (muscle fibers usually not rounded and hyaline fibers rare).
  5. Cardiac involvement less than in DMD.
  6. Occasionally linked with deuteranopia (color blindness).
  7. Mental retardation uncommon.
C. Limb-girdle dystrophy.
  1. Autosomal recessive (many sporadic); consanguineous mating increases incidence (first cousins, for example, have one-eighth of their genes in common).
  2. Onset usually in second or third decade.
  3. Life expectancy reduced but variable.

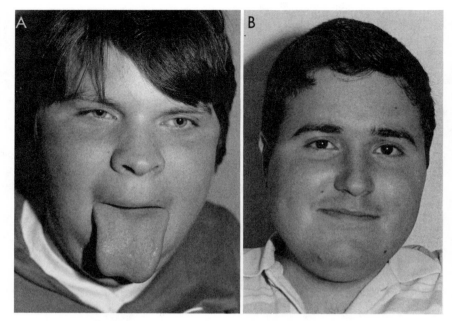

FIG 13–10.
A, macroglossia in DMD. B, masseter hypertrophy in DMD.

 a) Diaphragm involved early, which leads to alveolar hypoventilation.
 4. Limb-girdle (usually pelvic) weakness—variable progression. Prognosis is better in patients who manifest shoulder weakness first (Fig 13–11,A).
   a) Strong brachioradialis, sometimes marked atrophy of biceps.
   b) May have enlarged calves.
   c) Occasionally severe atrophy in periscapular muscles (Fig 13–11,B).
     (1) Upper extremities held in internal rotation during ambulation. May require thrown motion to move shoulder.
   d) Can have hypertrophy of extensor digitorum brevis.
   e) May find selective absence of a single muscle.
   f) "Popeye arms"—above elbow muscles atrophied, those below normal.
 5. No cardiomyopathy.

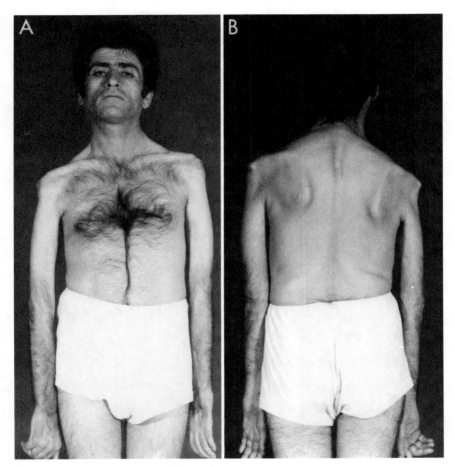

FIG 13–11.
LGD. **A,** frontal view. **B,** posterior view.

　6. Normal intelligence.
　7. Laboratory workup.
　　a) CPK modestly elevated.
　　b) EMG and biopsy myopathic.
　　c) Can be confused with Becker's dystrophy, Kugelberg-
　　　　Welander disease, metabolic myopathies, congenital
　　　　myopathies, polymyositis, and acid maltase deficiency.
　D. Facioscapulohumeral muscular dystrophy (Landouzy-
　　　Dejerine disease).

1. Autosomal dominant—full penetrance with variable expressivity (from patient to patient within a given pedigree, as well as from family to family). One parent always has at least subclinical disease.
2. Weakness of face, shoulder girdle (Fig 13–12,A) (particularly muscles of scapular fixation), anterior tibial muscles, hips, brachioradialis, and lower fibers of trapezius (Fig 13–12,B). Involvement usually asymmetrical in distribution and degree.
   a) Positive Bell's sign (Fig 13–13), accentuation of lateral lip "dimples," transverse smile, inability to whistle, wrinkle forehead or puff cheeks (Fig 13–14), "tapir" mouth (lip eversion and protrusion).

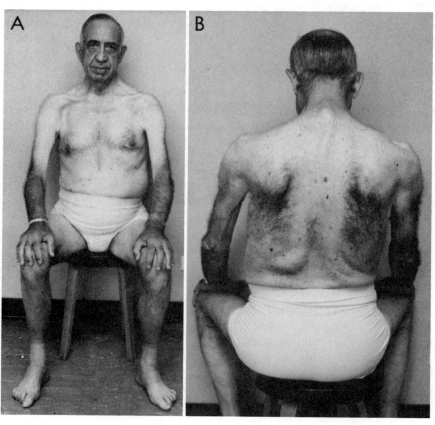

FIG 13–12.
FSH. **A,** frontal view. **B,** posterior view.

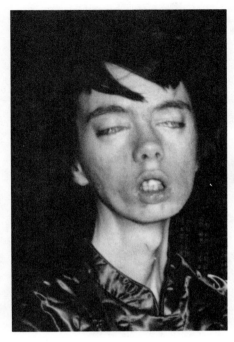

FIG 13–13.
FSH: Bell's sign.

   b) High riding scapulae.
   c) Foot drop—lower limbs usually affected 10–15 years after onset.
     (1) Distal leg weakness causes slapping gait.
   d) Deltoids often preserved.
   e) Increased lumbar lordosis.
   f) Dorsiflexor weakness of wrists and fingers ("praying mantis" posture) and toes. May be only apparent weakness (Fig 13–15).
   g) Pelvic girdle weakness with increased lumbar lordosis. Occasionally cauda equina syndrome with leg paresthesias secondary to sway back.
   h) Back extensors, quadriceps, and tensor fascia often exempt.
  3. Onset usually in adolescence or early adult life. Slow progression with normal life expectancy. May be stationary for periods of time.
   a) Childhood form is a more malign disease (Fig 13–16) (may show inflammatory response in muscle biopsy), running a more rapidly disabling course.

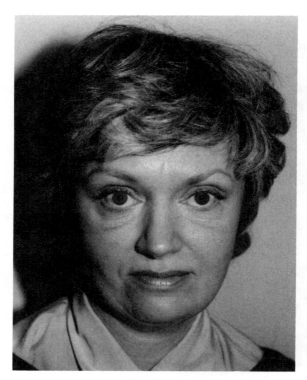

FIG 13–14.
FSH: facies.

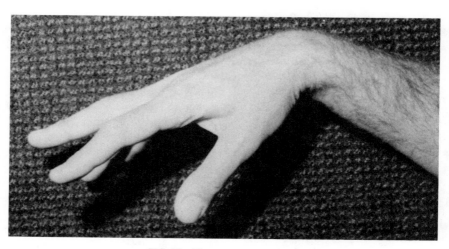

FIG 13–15.
FSH: wrist dorsiflexor weakness.

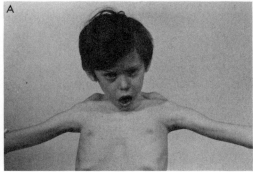

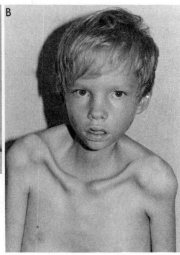

FIG 13–16.
FSH. **A** and **B**, childhood form.

4. Lab workup.
   a) CPK variably and slightly increased. Pyruvate kinase can be elevated (even when CPK normal).
   b) EMG myopathic but can show some neuropathic elements.
   c) Biopsy myopathic with an occasional inflammatory finding. Some cases show Type I fiber predominance.
5. Cardiac involvement and intellectual impairment not characteristic.

NOTE: Scapulo-peroneal muscular dystrophy (FSH minus the F)—muscle weakness mainly confined to these two groups of muscles. May be myopathic or neuropathic* (in which case EKG abnormalities are observed) and hereditary pattern is variable. X-linked disease can often be characterized as Emery-Dreifuss muscular dystrophy—insidious onset in childhood with Achilles tendon and elbow flexion contractures as well as inability to fully flex the neck and spine. Progression is slow without loss of ambulation. By mid-adulthood, atrial conduction defects occur that can cause sudden death.

The syndrome of facioscapulohumeral muscle weakness and wasting can be seen in such diverse conditions as myotubular myopathy, central core disease, nemaline myopathy, myasthenia gravis, poly-

---

*Almost every type of muscular dystrophy, except the X-linked or congenital diseases, seems to have a neurogenic counterpart.

myositis, adult acid-maltase deficiency, and spinal muscular atrophy. Figure 13–17 illustrates distribution of muscle weakness in DMD, LGD, and FSH.

 E. Ocular myopathies.
   1. Oculopharyngeal (Fig 13–18). Common in French Canadian families near Quebec and Spanish-American families in the southwestern United States. Regarded as a mitochondrial myopathy.
     a) Progressive (frequently asymmetrical) external ophthalmoplegia with dysphagia.
     b) Onset in third to fourth decade.
     c) Facial and limb muscles may be involved.
     d) CPK slightly increased, EMG myopathic.
     e) Usually autosomal dominant.
   2. Progressive ocular myopathy.
     a) Ptosis followed by ophthalmoplegia.
     b) Autosomal dominant or sporadic; women affected more than men.
     c) May have facial (and late upper limb) weakness.
     d) Usually begins in third decade.
     e) CPK normal, EMG myopathic, ragged red fibers on biopsy.
   3. Oculo-cranio-somatic neuromuscular disease (Fig 13–19).
     a) Progressive external ophthalmoplegia plus:
      (1) Retinitis pigmentosa and optic atrophy.

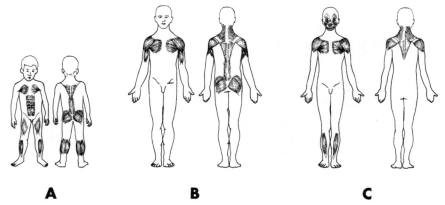

A   **B**   **C**

FIG 13–17.
Early distribution of muscle weakness in the three major forms of muscular dystrophy. **A,** Duchenne dystrophy. **B,** limb girdle dystrophy. **C,** facioscapulohumeral dystrophy.

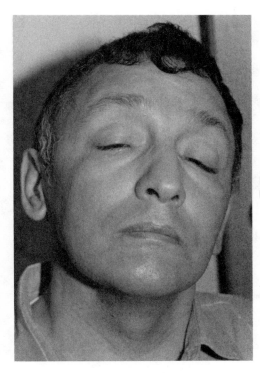

FIG 13–18.
Facies: oculopharyngeal dystrophy.

   (2) Cardiomyopathy and heart block.
   (3) Cerebellar ataxia and spasticity.
   (4) Deafness.
   (5) Mental retardation.
   (6) Skeletal deformities.
   (7) Limb myopathy.
   (8) Peripheral neuropathy.
   (9) Pharyngeal weakness.
  b) Onset in first several decades.
  c) CPK slightly elevated, EMG myopathic, ragged red fibers on biopsy.
 F. Distal myopathy.
  1. Inherited as a dominant character.
  2. Usually begins between 40–60 years of age.
  3. Affects small muscles of the hands and peripheral leg muscles with slow spread proximally.
  4. Comparatively benign condition found mostly in large Swedish kindreds.

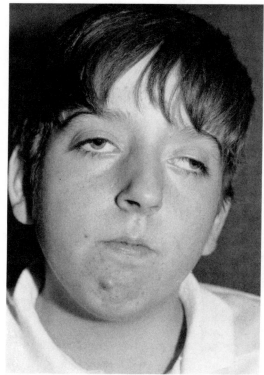

FIG 13–19.
External ophthalmoplegia.

G. Morphologically specific myopathies (so-called benign or congenital myopathies).
 1. Similar clinical picture for most types.
   a) Hypotonia after birth (floppy infants) or later occurring muscle weakness.
   b) Commonly slowly progressive generalized muscle weakness more marked proximally; facial or extraocular muscle weakness may be present. Occasionally rapid progression of disease.
   c) CPK usually normal.
   d) EMG normal or myopathic.
   e) Biopsy reveals specific identifying histological abnormality as seen by light or electron microscopy, and in many cases a Type I fiber predominance.
   f) Genetically determined (often autosomal dominant) but many sporadic cases.
   g) Can overlap with some of the metabolic myopathies.

h) Delayed motor milestones.
i) Skeletal abnormalities.
  (1) Congenital dislocation of the hip, particularly in central core disease.
    (a) Responds poorly to closed reduction because of muscle weakness. Usually requires operative stabilization.
  (2) Pes cavus.
  (3) Scoliosis.
j) Dysmorphic features.
  (1) High-arched palate.
  (2) Long-facies—dolichocephalic head.
  (3) Pectus carinatum or excavatum.
  (4) Absence of a single muscle (myotubular myopathy).
  (5) Long tapering fingers.
2. Major "structural" types—histological diagnosis.
  a) Central core disease.
  b) Nemaline myopathy (rod diseases)—childhood and adult forms.
  c) Myotubular myopathy.
  d) Mitochondrial myopathy.
  e) Multicore disease.
  f) Congenital fiber type disproportion.
H. Congenital muscular dystrophy.
  1. Hypotonia at birth (with facial involvement).
  2. Progressive muscular contractures.
  3. Usually no cardiomyopathy or intellectual impairment.
  4. Motor milestones met late but disease generally nonprogressive.
  5. CPK modestly elevated; EMG myopathic; biopsy shows advanced dystrophic changes with early and extensive endomysial fibrosis.
  6. Requires early aggressive orthopedic attention.
  7. Several kindreds with dysplastic brain abnormalities and dystrophic involvement of skeletal muscles have been reported in Japan (Fukuyama). These patients have markedly elevated CPK.

Metabolic Myopathies

Myopathies of varying severity, secondary to biochemical defects of muscle metabolism. May be progressive, fixed or recurrent, with exercise-induced weakness, cramps, and sometimes myoglobinuria. Diagnosis is made on the basis of clinical findings (e.g., an unusual craving for salt can be associated with one of the mitochondrial myopathies), enzyme assays, elevated CPK, EKG changes when heart is involved, typical histological findings (i.e., ragged red fibers in mitochondrial disease), EMG changes in some of the conditions, special histochemical staining to identify specific metabolites, or the lack of particular enzymes.

I. Glycogenosis. The seven recognized types of muscle disease associated with enzyme deficiency in the carbohydrate metabolism of muscle are outlined in Table 13–4. The site of action (liver, heart, muscle, etc.) of the deficient enzyme determines the format of the disease. Myopathy is present in Types II, III, V, and VII. In Types V and VII, myopathic symptoms are the major manifestation.

II. Abnormalities of lipid metabolism. Myopathies are characterized by neutral lipid accumulation in muscle due to mitochondrial metabolic defects. Carnitine (synthesized in the liver and transported via the blood stream) facilitates the passage of free fatty acids across the mitochondrial membrane. Diagnosis is by muscle biopsy (vacuolar [lipid] myopathy).

A. Carnitine deficiency.

1. Systemic: metabolic acidosis, encephalopathy, hepatomegaly, cardiomyopathy, and progressive muscular weakness.

2. Muscle: progressive proximal myopathy.

a) Can treat with diet (low in long-chain fatty acids), steroids, and oral L-carnitine.

3. Secondary to genetic defects of intermediary metabolism or other conditions (e.g., cytochrome oxidase deficiency, glutaric aciduria, chronic renal failure treated by hemodialysis, cirrhosis with cachexia, renal Fanconi syndrome).

B. Carnitine palmityl transferase deficiency. Postexertional or fasting pain with myoglobinuria, followed by weakness, tenderness, and muscle swelling. Treat with high carbohydrate foods or medium-chain fatty acid supplements.

III. Periodic paralyses. Episodic limb weakness usually occurring after exercise, typically spares muscles of respiration and disappears in an unpredictable manner. Clinical myotonia may be present. Tendency toward remission and relapse. Inherited as an autosomal dominant trait. Classified into hypokalemic, normokalemic, and hyperkalemic, depending on the level of venous blood potassium during an episode. These different forms may occur at different times in the same patient (biphasic periodic paralysis). Clinical

TABLE 13–4.
Glycogenoses

TYPE	ENZYME DEFICIENCY	EPONYMOUS OR OTHER NAMES	SKELETAL MUSCLE AFFECTED	CLINICAL FEATURES	OTHER TISSUES AFFECTED
I	Glucose-6-phosphatase	von Gierke's disease	No		Heart, nervous system kidneys, leucocytes
II	α-1,4-glucosidase (acid maltase)	Pompe's disease	Yes	(a) Severe form: generalized; resembles infantile spinal muscular atrophy (b) Mild form: resembles limb-girdle dystrophy, may present as adult	? Heart
III	Amylo-1,6-glucosidase ("debranching enzyme")	Limit dextrinosis Forbes' disease Cori's disease	Yes	Infantile hypotonia Mild weakness	Hepatic Hypoglycemia Ketosis Leucocytes
IV	α-1,4-glucan:α-1,4-glucan 6-glycosyl transferase ("branching enzyme"; amylo [1,4–1,6] transglucosidase)	Amylopectinosis Andersen's disease	? Some cases only	Usually no muscle symptoms In some wasting or weakness	Hepatomegaly Cirrhosis Splenomegaly
V	Muscle phosphorylase	McArdle's disease	Yes	Exercise intolerance Muscle cramps Fatigue Myoglobinuria Controlled with high glucose intake and avoiding strenuous activity	None
VI	Liver phosphorylase		No		
VII	Phosphofructokinase	Tarui's disease	Yes	Exercise intolerance Muscle cramps Fatigue, myoglobinuria	Erythrocytes

*From Dubowitz V: *Muscle Disorders in Childhood*. Philadelphia, WB Saunders Co, 1978. Used by permission.

features overlap. Provocative testing with potassium may be helpful in making the diagnosis. CPK can be raised during attacks. EMG changes may be present. Changes are apparent on biopsy if the specimen is taken during an attack. The primary defect for many of the periodic paralyses is believed to be an increased membrane conductance to sodium ions resulting in membrane hypoexcitability. Hypokalemic variety can often be induced by glucose and insulin, heavy exercise followed by rest, excessive alcohol, cold, trauma or stress, and can be treated with oral potassium, carbonic anhydrase inhibitors, sodium restriction, and high carbohydrate diet. Hyperkalemic paralysis can also be handled with acetazolamide as well as high carbohydrate intake. The normokalemic type is best relieved with sodium infusion. Carbonic anhydrase inhibitors may also help. Table 13–5 lists differential diagnosis of episodic weakness.

Malignant Hyperthermia

This is a syndrome initiated by a hypermetabolic state of skeletal muscle and characterized by rapid and sustained temperature rise during general anesthesia (surgical stress), accompanied by tachycardia, tachypnea, muscular rigidity, cyanosis, and severe metabolic and respiratory acidosis. Total body consumption of oxygen increases to two to three times normal and temperature can rise (as fast as 1°C every five minutes) to as high as 43°C. Serum CPK and potassium are markedly elevated. Muscle necrosis follows with myoglobinuria and sometimes renal shutdown.

I. Usually expressed as an autosomal dominant trait, but inheritance may be multifactorial. Patients with myopathy (including DMD and DMD carriers) are at increased risk, particularly central core disease.

TABLE 13–5.
Causes of Episodic Weakness*

1. Periodic paralysis
2. Relapsing polyneuropathy
3. Dermatomyositis; polymyositis
4. Myasthenia gravis
5. Rhabdomyolysis

*From Dubowitz V: *Muscle Disorders in Childhood.* Philadelphia, WB Saunders Co, 1978. Used by permission.

A. It is important to look for a history of similar problems with anesthesia in the family.
B. Patients may have large muscle mass (they tend to be muscular and athletic) and a history of cramping (especially nocturnal, which tends to stop by the third decade), exercise intolerance in hot weather, and stress-associated acrocyanosis. Musculoskeletal abnormalities such as ptosis, clubfoot, scoliosis, pectus carinatum, and hernia are common.

II. Incidence 1:15,000 anesthetics in children; 1:50,000 in adults. Sexes affected equally in childhood; most postpubescent victims are males.
A. Attacks may not necessarily occur with the first exposure to general anesthesia.

III. Elevated CPK may be found during workup.

IV. Mild myopathic changes present in some patients.

V. Halothane and succinylcholine are the most provocative anesthetic agents, although any general anesthetic can cause an incident.
A. If local or regional anesthesia is not feasible, general anesthesia can be accomplished with nitrous oxide, narcotics, barbiturates, ketamine, or droperidol.

VI. Muscle biopsy shows abnormal in vitro sensitivity to halothane, succinylcholine, or caffeine, which increase calcium efflux into the cell.
A. The marked elevation of temperature is believed to be secondary to high calcium concentration in the myoplasm.

VII. Treatment.
A. Stop anesthesia and administer 100% oxygen.
B. Cool the patient externally and internally (gastric, rectal, peritoneal lavage) to combat hyperthermia.
C. Insert bladder and CVP catheters.
D. Administer:
   1. Intravenous procaine or procainamide (avoid lidocaine) to combat rigidity. These drugs decrease intracellular calcium transport.
   2. Intravenous steroids.
   3. Bicarbonate to control metabolic acidosis.
   4. Glucose and insulin infusion to treat hyperkalemia.
   5. Dantrolene sodium (I.V.—2.5 to 10.0 mg/kg) may abort an attack. Action: Excitation-contraction uncoupling by decreasing release of calcium from sarcoplasmic reticulum.
      a) Preanesthetic oral dantrolene loading (4–8 mg/kg for

two days with final dose two hours before anesthesia)
may abort or lessen the severity of an episode.
E. Monitor for renal failure after recovery.

Myotonic Disorders

This is a group of conditions (usually hereditary) having in common
clinical myotonia (delay of muscular relaxation after contraction). This
is best seen in the clenched fist or in the orbicularis oculi muscles.
Myotonia in all myotonic diseases is often aggravated by cold. It can
be improved (fatigues) by repetitive activities, but sometime this increases its severity (myotonia paradoxica). Myotonia can be elicited by
percussion. This is usually demonstrated in the tongue or thenar muscles. EMG is characterized by high-frequency repetitive discharges that
initially increase in frequency and amplitude and then rapidly diminish
(dive-bomber effect). Myotonia is of muscular origin and independent
of motor nerve activity. The repetitive electrical activity persists even
though the motor nerve is sectioned or the neuromuscular junction
blocked with curare. It is believed to be a membrane defect (hyperex-
citability) related to an abnormality of chloride (myotonia congenita) or
calcium (dystrophia myotonica) conductance. It can be induced by
drugs (i.e., clofibrate), may appear as a remote effect of lung carcinoma, may be found in thyroid dysfunction or adult acid maltase deficiency. The major forms of myotonic disease are:

I. Myotonia congenita (Thomsen's disease).
   A. Generalized nonprogressive muscular hypertrophy with mus-
      cle stiffness and weakness, relieved by exercise, occurring in
      two forms.
      1. Autosomal dominant; mild nonprogressive myotonia diag-
         nosed in infancy.
      2. Autosomal recessive; later onset with subsequent distal
         atrophy and weakness.
   B. EMG myotonic; CPK slightly elevated; biopsy fiber hypertro-
      phy. Increased creatine tolerance.
   C. May present with complaint of garbled speech after eating
      iced foods (associated with tongue myotonia induced by cold).
II. Dystrophia myotonica (Steinert's disease).
   A. An autosomal dominant multisystem disorder (linked with the
      secretor gene) with poor congruence in affected family mem-
      bers, the commonest form of which usually becomes apparent

in early adulthood. Expression is variable, and the disease is characterized by:
1. Stellate cataracts and retinal alterations.
2. Gonadal atrophy.
   a) Impotence in males, chronic abortion in females.
3. Faulty tolerance to carbohydrate (diabetic glucose tolerance curve). Defective insulin metabolism.
   a) Mild (end organ) "diabetes" is common to many muscle diseases.
4. EKG abnormalities.
5. Frontal and parietal alopecia in males.
6. Thyroid dysfunction.
7. Low IgG level (hypercatabolized); low urinary creatinine; may have low serum uric acid.
8. Cardiac conduction defects sometimes requiring demand pacemakers. Stokes-Adams attacks are common.
9. Impaired pulmonary function. Pickwickian syndrome. Alveolar hypoventilation (night sweats, nightmares).
10. Progressive psychosocial deterioration with fall-off of higher intellectual functions. Paranoid tendency. "Belle indifference," "whining dependence" and depression (which may respond to tricyclic antidepressant treatment).
11. Low basal metabolic rate.
12. Cerebral ventricular dilatation.
13. Skull abnormalities, including hyperostosis cranii, decrease in sella turcica size, prognathism, hyperostosis frontalis interna, and enlargement of the paranasal sinuses.
14. Lugubrious facies with ptosis. Thin, haggard, expressionless face. Transverse smile, hollow temples and cheeks (Fig 13–20). Sternocleidomastoid (particularly clavicular head) (Fig 13–21) weakening, leading to "swan neck."
15. Temporal muscle wasting; myotonic lid lag.
16. Distal muscle weakness, especially in the forearms and tibialis anterior muscles. Patient may trip because of weakness, and in attempting to regain balance, provoke a myotonic response that causes a fall. It is the weakness (dystrophy), not the myotonia, that troubles these patients the most.
17. Percussion and effort myotonia.
    a) Hand (slowness in grip release).

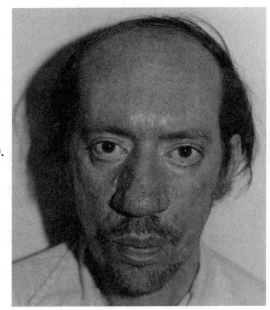

FIG 13–20.
DM: facies.

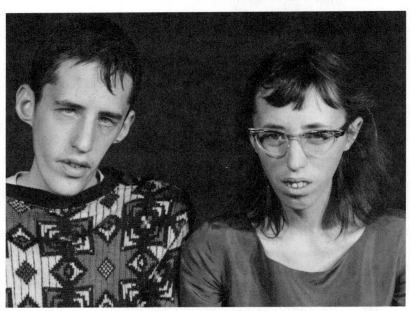

FIG 13–21.
DM: early onset in siblings.

b) Tongue (dimpling on percussion).
c) Thenar eminence (contracture on percussion) (Fig 13–22).
d) Spasm of globe elevators (after forced eyelid closure with sudden release).

NOTE: Myotonia persists after nerve section, block, or curarization. It is increased by cold, fatigue, or sudden stress. It tends to lessen and sometimes disappear in the later stages of the disease as muscular weakness advances.

18. Dysphagia (late) because of pharyngeal myotonia and dysarthria secondary to tongue myotonia.
19. Smooth muscle disorders of lower GI tract (megacolon).
20. Increased incidence of gallbladder disease.
21. Sometimes a high-frequency hearing defect.
22. Neuronal heterotopias.
23. Nasal speech (because of pharyngeal muscle weakness).
24. CPK may be slightly elevated; EMG myotonic; nerve conduction (motor and sensory) may be slowed; muscle biopsy—many internal nuclei appearing in long chains on longitudinal section, sarcoplasmic masses, ring fibers, selective Type I fiber atrophy.

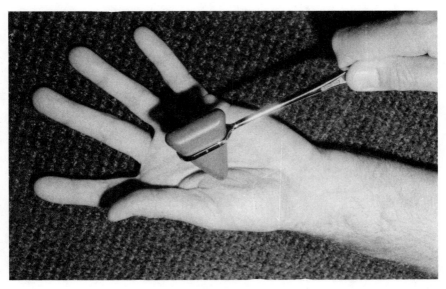

FIG 13–22.
Percussion myotonia.

TABLE 13–6.
A Working Classification of the Common Diseases of Muscle*

TYPE†	AGE OF ONSET	SEX	SYMPTOMS	COURSE	MISCELLANEOUS
Childhood dystrophy Severe (Duchenne) Benign (Becker) Later onset, slower progression	1 to 4 years	Male, primarily	Clumsiness, toewalking, lordosis, Gowers' sign, pseudohypertrophy	Increasing weakness with contracture, wheelchair by age 8 to 10, death in late teens	Mental retardation—30%–50% abnormal EKG—50%
Limb-girdle dystrophy	Any; commonly 2nd to 3rd decade	Equal	Extensor weakness, shoulders and hips	Slow progress with late disability	Occasional pseudohypertrophy
Facioscapulohumeral dystrophy (Landouzy Dejerine)	2nd to 4th decade‡	Equal	Paucity of facial expression, variable speech defect, difficulty in abducting arms, scapular winging, Bell's sign	Progressive weakness, very late disability	Variable life expectancy; little tendency to develop contractures
Dystrophia myotonica	Adult life‡	Equal	Myotonia, lugubrious facies, severe fatigability, dropfoot gait	Slowly progressive weakness, temporal baldness, cataracts, gonadal atrophy, sterility, impotence, hypothyroidism, diabetes, acromegaly, hyperostosis cranii	Mildly progressive social and mental retardation

*Adapted from Coodley EL (ed): *Diagnostic Enzymology*. Philadelphia, Lea & Febiger, p 262.
†Approximately one-third of all cases of muscular dystrophy occur sporadically. Other, less common types include the ophthalmoplegic form, distal myopathy, central core disease, arthrogryposis. McArdle's syndrome and nemaline (rod) myopathy. Two distinct types of dystrophy in one family have never been reported.
‡Can present in childhood.

Table 13–6 presents a working outline of the common diseases of muscle (DMD, LGD, FSH, DM).
B. Treatment of myotonia.*
   1. Phenytoin, 100 mg t.i.d., decreases sodium influx during membrane excitation.
   2. Acetazolamide, 125–500 mg/day, promotes mild kaluresis rendering muscle more resistant to depolarization.
   3. Quinine, grains 5 t.i.d., stabilizes membrane.
   4. Procainamide, 0.5 to 1.0 g q.i.d., stabilizes muscle membrane but may impair cardiac conduction and can cause a lupus-like syndrome.
   5. Steroids.
C. Congenital (neonatal) dystrophia myotonica.
   1. Severe generalized hypotonia at birth.
   2. Facial diplegia with sucking and breathing difficulty.
   3. Bilateral talipes requiring early and vigorous orthopedic attention (Fig 13–23).
   4. Frequent hydramnios in mother.
   5. Mental retardation.
   6. Electrical and mechanical myotonia observed later.
   7. Characteristic inverted V configuration to upper lip (shark mouth) (Fig 13–24).
   8. Dysmaturation almost always inherited from myotonic mother.
   9. Muscle biopsy—maturational arrest at various fetal developmental stages
III. Paramyotonia congenita (VanEulenberg).
   A. Autosomal dominant condition manifest at birth by mild myotonia of face and hands, aggravated by cold, with tendency to muscle hypertrophy. May be due to temperature-dependent abnormality in sodium conductance.
   B. Patient's muscle stiffness may be increased or reduced by exercise.
   C. May suffer episodes of flaccid weakness similar to the periodic paralyses.

*Ethyl alcohol can decrease myotonia, but no case of an alcoholic myotonic has yet been reported. Quinine, in addition to causing tinnitus at high doses, has an adverse cardiac effect. Procainamide can cause lupus and also slows cardiac conduction. The side effects of phenytoin include gingival hyperplasia, nystagmus, GI upset, pseudolymphoma, blood dyscrasias, SLE-like syndrome, dysarthria, ataxia, hirsutism, skin rash, and osteomalacia. Most drugs effective in reducing myotonia are membrane stabilizers.

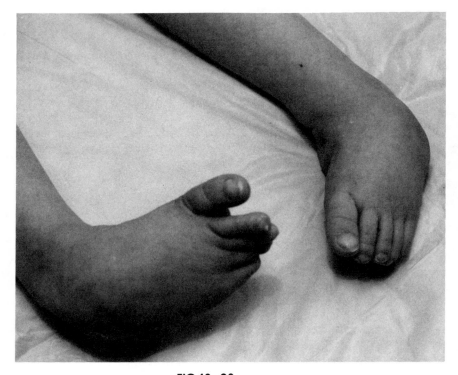

FIG 13—23.
Neonatal DM: talipes.

    D. Lid lag may be elicited (also found in myotonia congenita and in hyperthyroid myopathy).

    NOTE: Clinical myotonia as an ancillary sign may be found in Schwartz-Jampel syndrome. It can also be seen in myxedema, hypokalemic paralysis, and after treatment with a variety of drugs interfering with muscle membrane lipid metabolism. Electrical myotonia may be noted in acid maltase deficiency and denervation.

Endocrine Myopathies

Myopathy can accompany a variety of endocrine disorders. These usually occur in adults. The onset of weakness is insidious. Proximal muscles are predominantly affected. CPK is elevated, creatinuria is present, and the EMG shows myopathic characteristics. However, there may be

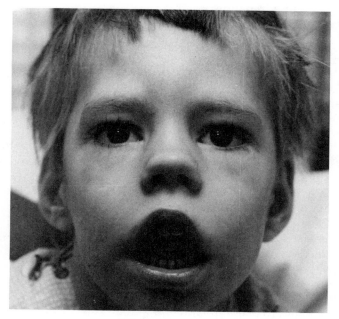

FIG 13–24.
Neonatal DM: facies.

indications of neuropathic causation. Management of the primary disorder consists of organ-specific treatment.

I. Thyroid myopathies.
  A. Hyperthyroidism.
    1. Bulbar and EOM can be involved in severe thyrotoxicosis (this may be myasthenic). Lid lag may be seen.
  B. Hypothyroidism.
    1. Muscle spasm and cramps can occur.
    2. Delayed relaxation of ankle reflex.
    3. May find electrical myotonia.
II. Parathyroid disorders.
  A. Hypoparathyroidism.
    1. Tetany with carpopedal spasm.
  B. Hyperparathyroidism and osteomalacia.
    1. Proximal weakness.
    2. Muscle tenderness and aching.
    3. EMG signs of denervation.

III. Pituitary and adrenal disorders.
   A. Hypoadrenalism (Addison's disease).
      1. Fatigability and muscle cramping.
      2. Proximal wasting.
      3. Periodic episodes of hypokalemic weakness.
   B. Hyperadrenalism (Cushing's syndrome).
      1. Proximal weakness and wasting of insidious onset.
IV. Steroid myopathy. This nonspecific proximal muscle weakness is seen with the administration of steroids, especially the halogenated compounds (e.g., triamcinolone (Fig 13–25), dexamethasone). May be due in part to epinephrine suppression, which blocks phosphorylase activation. Can prove difficult to diagnose, especially in the case of an inflammatory myopathy under treatment with glucocorticoids.
   A. CPK may be normal.
   B. Increased creatinuria (in presence of normal or low serum enzyme level).
   C. EMG—short-duration polyphasic motor unit action potentials.
   D. Type II atrophy on biopsy (versus inflammatory necrosis in polymyositis).
   E. Weakness (usually in large antigravity postural muscles of lower extremities) may be dose related and develop rapidly.
   F. Muscles often tender to palpation.
   G. Other signs of hypersteroidism commonly present:
      1. Moon facies.
      2. Increase in adipose tissue.
      3. Acne vulgaris, diabetes.

FIG 13–25.
Triamcinolone.

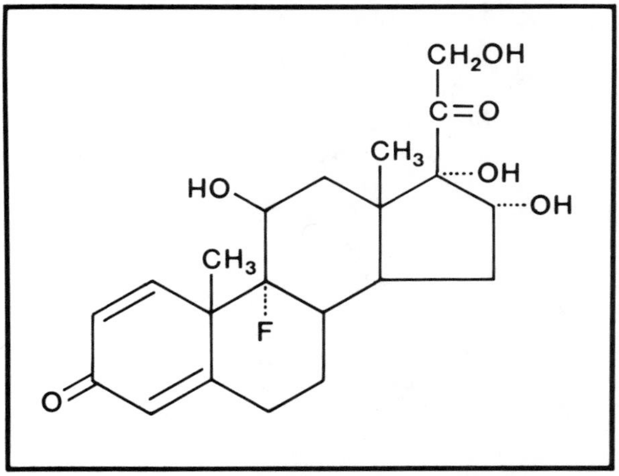

4. Osteoporosis (with vertebral compression fracture).
5. Hypertension, psychiatric disorders.
H. Improvement with discontinuation of steroid medication.
V. Acromegaly.
   A. Early muscle hypertrophy followed by late proximal weakness.
VI. Hyperaldosteronism.
   A. Periodic attacks of hypokalemic weakness.

Nutritional and Drug-Induced Myopathies

I. Protein deprivation.
II. Osteomalacia.
III. Alcoholic myopathy.
   A. Acute.
      1. After heavy drinking bout.
      2. Sudden onset of muscle pain with swelling and weakness, typically in the large appendicular postural muscles. CPK markedly elevated (even modest alcoholic intake causes some increase in serum CPK).
      3. Muscle can be swollen and tender.
      4. Necrotizing myopathy (selective Type II atrophy with excess lipid and glycogen in fibers suggesting a metabolic pathway inhibition) resulting in:
         a) Myoglobinuria.
         b) Renal failure which requires supportive treatment.
   B. Chronic.
      1. Slowly progressive limb-girdle weakness. Most of the effects of chronic alcoholism are due to vitamin deficiencies, particularly of vitamin B_1.
IV. Other drugs that can cause neuromuscular pathology.
   A. Vincristine—weakness.
   B. Diazacholesterol—myotonia.
   C. Clofibrate—cramping.
   D. Penicillamine—inflammatory myopathy.
   E. Diuretics, licorice, purgatives—hypokalemic paralysis.
   F. Chloroquine, heroin—subacute painless myopathy.
   G. Cimetidine, lithium—mild weakness.

Inflammatory Myopathies

These disorders are thought to be due to a viral or autoimmune mechanism and are characterized by symmetrical proximal muscle weakness often accompanied by muscular pain and tenderness.* They occur more frequently in blacks. Dysphagia is sometimes present. Involvement of the facial or EOM is rare. Pseudohypertrophy occasionally occurs. The deep tendon reflexes may be absent, normal, or hyperactive. The heart can be involved. Muscle atrophy with contracture and calcinosis† are seen late in the course of the disease. CPK is raised as well as ESR and WBC (50% of cases). Elevated ANA, positive latex test (50%), and increase in serum gamma globulins α_2, and IgM have also been reported. EMG shows polyphasic, brief, small motor action potentials with spontaneous fibrillations and positive sharp waves, insertional irritability, and bizarre high-frequency repetitive discharges. Muscle pathology includes inflammatory cellular infiltrates (principally lymphocytes), segmental necrosis, de- and regeneration (necrosis, vacuolization and phagocytosis), and increase of endomysial connective tissue. Perifascicular atrophy of both Type I and II fibers is present. This pattern is probably related to ischemic myopathy of fibers adjacent to perimysial collagenous septae and is more common in dermatomyositis. All of these biopsy findings are usually scattered.

Polymyositis is the diagnostic label given a nonhereditary inflammatory myopathy. Where a skin rash is present, the term *dermatomyositis* is used. These conditions can present acutely or run a subacute, relapsing, or chronic course. There are both childhood and adult forms. A bimodal age distribution, between ages 5 and 15 and then between 50 and 60 years, has been reported. Polymyositis is as common as scleroderma, and half as common as systemic lupus erythematosus. Its incidence is five to eight new cases per million people each year. Inflammatory myopathy in childhood can be confused with DMD. The differential diagnosis is outlined in Table 13–7.

I. Idiopathic polymyositis.
   A. Pain and stiffness more marked in upper limbs, weakness in lower, but one-third of patients present with a nonmuscular first symptom. May also mimic DMD almost completely.
   B. Cervical flexors involved early.
   C. Dysphagia, dysphonia, arthralgia, and Raynaud's phenomenon may occur. Arthritis, usually of the hands, may occur in patients with chronic disease. Instability of the thumb at the interphalangeal joint may require fusion.
   D. Systemic symptoms (fever, weight loss, lethargy) are common.

*Myalgia in the absence of weakness betokens other disorders, such as vascular disease, polymyalgia rheumatica, or hypothyroidism.
†The development of such calcinosis, usually manifest in childhood dermatomyositis, is unaffected by treatment with steroids.

TABLE 13–7.
Differential Diagnosis*

CATEGORY	POLYMYOSITIS	MUSCULAR DYSTROPHY (DUCHENNE)
Age of onset	Any	Usually 2–6 years
Sex	Females, males	Males
Genetic transmission	None	Sex-linked recessive
Clinical signs and symptoms	Walk at normal age, then develop muscle weakness	Late walkers, begin to stumble, fall, have difficulty climbing stairs
Pseudohypertrophy	May occur	Occurs in 80%
Deep tendon reflexes	May be absent, normal, or hyperactive	Gradual loss except at ankles
Course	Variable; may have slow or rapid deterioration with exacerbations and remissions	Steady progression with confinement to wheelchair usually in second decade
Life span	May be shortened	20–25 years
Treatment	Prednisone 75 mg/m-2; physical therapy	Physical therapy; night casts, braces
Pathology	Infiltration of round cells; areas of regeneration	Fatty infiltration; central migration of sarcolemmal nuclei; fibrosis

*From Thompson CE: Polymyositis in children, in *Clinical Pediatrics*, vol 7. Philadelphia, JB Lippincott Co, 1968. Used by permission.

    E. Cardiac involvement has been reported.
 II. Idiopathic dermatomyositis (Fig 13–26).
    A. Female:male ratio 2:1.
    B. Less common than polymyositis in adults.
    C. More malign disease than polymyositis.
    D. Myopathy similar to polymyositis but rash present.
      1. Violaceous butterfly facial distribution (Fig 13–27).
      2. Heliotrope rash of eyelids.
      3. Periorbital edema.
      4. Erythema, scaly rash, or telangiectasia of forehead, neck, shoulder, chest, back, elbows or knees. Gottron's papules on the knuckles.
      5. Late skin and subcutaneous nodular calcifications, mostly in children and correlated with a favorable outcome.
    E. Childhood type.
      1. Not associated with neoplasm.
      2. Skin lesions can be florid or minimal.
      3. Severe malaise and listlessness.
      4. Usually insidious onset.

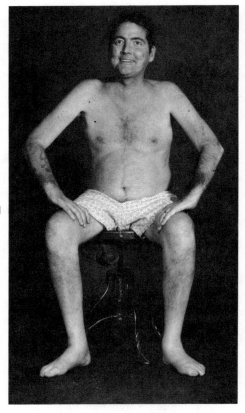

FIG 13–26.
Distribution of atrophy, rash, and edema in dermatomyositis.

  5. Systemic involvement.
     a) Arthralgia; also, calcinosis of subcutaneous tissue and
        interstitial tissues of muscle (Fig 13–28).
     b) Hepato- and splenomegaly.
     c) Pneumonitis—pulmonary fibrosis.
     d) GI ulcerations secondary to vasculitis.
     e) Cardiac involvement.
     f) Renal involvement.
     g) Necrosing vasculitis and other angiopathic features.
     h) Muscular contractures.
  6. C-reactive protein normal (elevated with infection); CPK
     may be normal.
III. Polymyositis and collagen vascular disease. Both dermatomyositis
     and polymyositis may complicate other connective tissue disor-

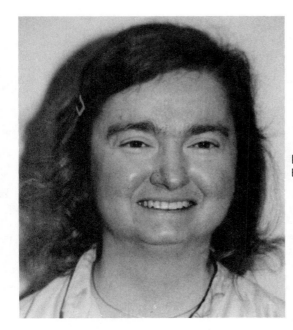

FIG 13–27.
Butterfly facial rash.

ders ("overlap syndrome"). Either may be found in association
with:
  A. Rheumatoid arthritis.
  B. Systemic lupus erythematosus.
  C. Scleroderma.
  D. Periarteritis nodosa.
IV. Inflammatory myositis associated with neoplasm.
  A. Many autoimmune diseases are associated with an increased
      incidence of neoplasia. Dermatomyositis with onset after 40
      years of age (particularly in a male) is often accompanied by a
      malignant disease.
  B. All types of malignancy may occur. Carcinoma of lung, breast,
      ovary, uterus, prostate, and stomach are most frequent.
  C. In most cases, the manifestations of inflammatory myopathy
      precede those of the tumor.
  D. Treatment of the neoplasm may have a favorable effect on as-
      sociated muscle and skin lesions.
  V. Miscellaneous diseases that can cause secondary inflammatory
      myopathy.
  A. Polymyalgia rheumatica.
  B. Eosinophilic fasciitis.

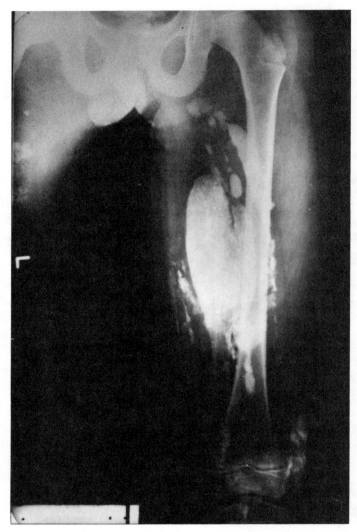

FIG 13–28.
Soft tissue calcification in childhood dermatomyositis.

    C. Trichinosis.
    D. Sarcoid.
     E. Cysticercosis.
  VI. Treatment.
    A. Steroids.

1. High doses for three months.
   a) Avoid fluorinated steroids (dexamethasone and triamcinolone) as they more frequently induce steroid myopathy.
   b) Adults: 50–100 mg/kg/day.
   c) Children: 1–2 mg/kg/day.
2. Schedule.
   a) Initial daily dose.
   b) Can switch to alternate-day dosage two to four weeks after initiating treatment.
   c) Observe patient closely for complications.
       (1) Acute.
           (a) Edema.
           (b) Weight gain.
           (c) Hypertension.
           (d) Diabetes.
           (e) GI hemorrhage.
       (2) Chronic.
           (a) Cataracts and ocular hypertension.
           (b) Infection and poor wound healing.
           (c) Psychosis.
           (d) Osteoporosis (fractures).
           (e) Delayed growth.
           (f) Myopathy.
           (g) Cushinoid features.
               i) Moon facies.
               ii) Central obesity.
               iii) Buffalo hump.
               iv) Facial hirsutism.
               v) Abdominal and thigh striae.
           (h) Spontaneous tendon ruptures.
           (i) Acne and thinning of skin.
   d) Necessary adjuncts to steroid therapy include:
       (1) Low-sodium, high-potassium intake.
       (2) Antacids.
       (3) High-protein, low-carbohydrate diet.
   e) Can reduce dose when clinical response has occurred.
       (1) Reduce very slowly.
       (2) Titrate treatment with serial CPK determinations, but remember that CPK normalization or increase may precede clinical remission or reacerbation by at least several weeks. EMG can also be used to monitor dis-

ease activity (fibrillation potentials indicate active disease).

(3) Increase dose slightly or return to daily dosage if symptoms worsen or CPK increases.

f) Recovery from dermatomyositis or polymyositis is slow (although spontaneous remissions can occur) and, although some patients recover completely (the overall survival rate of both treated and untreated patients is 80% after five years, although treatment seems to improve strength and lessen discomfort), minimal supportive steroid treatment may be necessary for years in others. However, in children, tapering of the dose can usually begin earlier (persistence of skin rash is not indicative of active disease), and steroid treatment can often be discontinued within three to six months.

B. Immunosuppressive drugs.
   1. Initiate when no response to three to six months of steroid treatment. These drugs have potential teratogenic effects.
      a) Methotrexate, 15–30 mg/day, may cause severe ulcerative stomatitis and leukopenia.
      b) Azathioprine, 3 mg/kg/day, can cause drug fever.
      c) Cyclophosphamide, 2 mg/kg/day, may produce hemorrhagic cystitis.
   2. Plasmapheresis has been used as an adjutant to immunosuppressive therapy.
C. Other measures.
   1. Physical therapy to prevent or treat contractures.
   2. Night splints as indicated.
   3. Topical steroids and Burow's solution soaks for skin lesions.
   4. Diphosphonates for calcinosis in dermatomyositis.
D. Factors decreasing survivorship (most deaths occur in the first two years after diagnosis).
   1. Age greater than 50 years.
   2. Black race.
   3. Extreme weakness—dysphagia.
   4. Pneumonitis.
   5. Neoplasm.
   6. Associated collagen disease.

MISCELLANEOUS

I. Prader-Willi syndrome (H_3O syndrome—hypotonia, hypomentia, hypogonadism, obesity). Chromosome 15 breakage/translocation has been demonstrated in several cases.
   A. Patients present with typical appearance of fair hair, blue eyes, high forehead, and small, almond-shaped eyes.
   B. Diabetes develops in adolescence.
   C. CPK, EMG, and biopsy are all normal.
   D. Higher incidence in males.
   E. Marked hypotonia at birth—floppy infant.
   F. Compulsive eating beginning in early childhood.
II. Arthrogryposis (curved joints).
   A. Symptom-complex, not a specific diagnostic entity.
   B. Characterized by multiple joint contractures secondary to immobility of limbs in utero.
   C. May be myopathic or neuropathic.
   D. Must differentiate from congenital muscular dystrophy and spinal muscular atrophy.
   E. Joint rigidity is secondary to fibrous ankylosis.
   F. Fixed deformities can be surgically improved by aggressive soft tissue release.
III. Stiff man syndrome.
   A. Sustained repetitive activity of muscle fibers affecting both sexes, usually in adult life.
      1. May be preceded by pain and tightness of back and chest muscles.
      2. Results in uncontrollable contractions, mostly of musculature of the limb girdles, but any and all voluntary muscles may become involved.
      3. Dyspnea, dysphagia, and facial grimacing can occur.
      4. The limbs are held in rigid distorted positions and the spasms are painful.
      5. Stiffness disappears during sleep (EEG shows less REM sleep than normal) and general anesthesia, and may be elicited by a variety of stimuli (active or passive movement, emotional stress).
   B. Physical examination reveals occasional hyperreflexia and extensor plantar responses.
   C. EMG shows a sustained interference pattern but is otherwise normal.

    D. Muscle spasms are abolished by curare peripheral nerve block and spinal anesthesia.

    E. Proposed etiology.

        1. Gamma system overactivity.

        2. Lack of normal inhibitory feedback to anterior horn cells.

        3. Catecholaminergic—GABA system imbalance.

    F. Treatment—high-dose diazepam (up to 300 mg/day) or baclofen.

    NOTE: Neuromyotonia (continuous muscle fiber activity) is yet another condition of abnormal muscle activity. It is characterized by myokymia secondary to brief tetanic contractions of muscle fibers. This can be diagnosed by EMG. It may be simply annoying or severe enough to cause rigidity and deformity. Pathology is apparently in the peripheral nerve. Treatment is with diphenylhydantoin or carbamazepine.

  IV. Inclusion body myositis.

    A. Progressive painless limb-girdle weakness.

    B. Normal or mildly elevated CPK.

    C. Unresponsive to steroids or immunosuppressive drugs.

    D. Biopsy.

        1. Myopathic changes.

        2. Mononuclear inflammatory infiltrates.

        3. Vacuoles lined with basophilic granules in muscle fibers.

  V. Myopathy may attend a variety of other diseases such as the col-

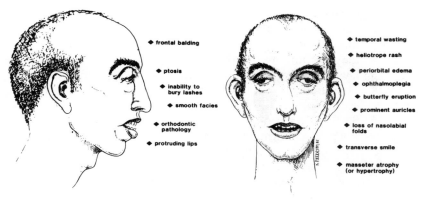

FIG 13–29.
Some common facial alterations in neuromuscular disease. (From Siegel I: The many faces of neuromuscular disease. *Postgrad Med* 1986; 7:121–137. Used by permission.)

TABLE 13-8.

Classification of Neuromuscular Disorders by Usual Age of Patient at Clinical Presentation

Birth-Infancy
  HMSN III
  Neonatal myasthenia gravis
  Morphologically specific (congenital) myopathies
  Glycogenosis
  Lipid myopathies
  Myotonia congenita
  Neonatal dystrophia myotonica
  Arthrogryposis

Early Childhood (usually progressive)
  DMD
  Prader-Willi syndrome
  HMSN IV
  HMSN V
  Juvenile myasthenia gravis
  FSH-childhood form
  Oculo-cranio-somatic neuromuscular disease
  Some glycogen-storage diseases

Late Childhood-Adolescence (often progressive)
  HMSN I
  Becker's dystrophy
  Limb-girdle dystrophy
  Periodic paralyses
  Some cases of myotonia congenita

Adulthood
  HMSN II
  ALS
  Some cases of LGD
  FSH
  Myasthenia gravis
  Ocular myopathy
  Distal myopathy
  Dystrophia myotonica
  Paramyotonia congenita
  Stiff man syndrome
  Sarcoid myopathy

Onset at Any Age
  SMA
  Poliomyelitis
  Acquired neuropathies
  Endocrine myopathies (usually adulthood)
  Nutritional or drug-induced myopathies
  Inflammatory myopathies (dermatomyositis often in childhood)

lagen vascular disorders (LE, rheumatoid arthritis, polyarteritis nodosa), sarcoid, carcinoma, Marfan's syndrome.

Figures 13–29 and Tables 13–8 to 13–13 summarize various features of diagnosis and classification of muscle disease.

TABLE 13–9.

Classification of Neuromuscular Disorders by Usual Major Site of Involvement

Proximal Muscle Groups
  Myasthenia gravis
  DMD
  LGD
  Becker's dystrophy
  FSH
  Ocular myopathy
  Steroid myopathy
  Hyperthyroidism
  Hyperparathyroidism
  Hyperadrenalism
  Acromegaly
  Alcoholic myopathy
  Inflammatory myopathies
  Sarcoid myopathy

Distal Muscle Groups
  Charcot-Marie-Tooth disease
  Distal myopathy
  Dystrophia myotonica
  Peripheral motor neuropathies

Either Proximal, Distal, or Both Muscle Groups
  SMA
  ALS
  Poliomyelitis
  Refsum's disease
  Dejerine-Sottas
  Friedreich's ataxia
  Oculo-cranio-somatic disease
  Morphologically specific (congenital) myopathies
  Glycogenosis
  Carnitine deficiency
  Periodic paralysis
  Neonatal dystrophia myotonica
  Myotonia congenita

TABLE 13–10.
Some Diseases Displaying Myotonia on EMG Examination

Myotonia congenita (Thomsen's disease)
Dystrophia myotonica (Steinert's disease)
Paramyotonia congenita (van
   Eulenberg)
Schwartz-Jampel syndrome
Periodic paralysis (hyperkalemic)
Acid-maltase deficiency
Inflammatory myopathy
Hyperthyroidism
Drugs
   20,25-diazocholesterol
   Monocarboxylic aromatic acids
   2,4-dihydroxy acetate
   Clofibrate
   Triparonol

TABLE 13–11.
Some Conditions Showing Predominantly Distal Limb Wasting

Hereditary sensory and motor neuropathy
Motor neuron disease
Acquired neuropathies
Dystrophia myotonica
Distal myopathy
Nemaline rod disease
Scapuloperoneal dystrophy

TABLE 13–12.
Differential Diagnosis, Pathology, and Treatment of Some Common Causes of Acute Onset of Muscle Weakness

DISEASE	SEEN IN	HISTORY	EXAMINATION (POSITIVE FINDINGS)	LAB (POSITIVE FINDINGS)	PATHOPHYSIOLOGY	TREATMENT
Myasthenia gravis	Young F Older M	Fatigue; improved with rest Bulbar symptoms	Ptosis EOM weakness Difficulty chewing Dysphagia Dysarthria Myopathic facies Appendicular fatigue	EMG-decremental response Acetylcholinesterase antibody receptor decrease Positive tension test	Blockage of acetylcholine receptors at neuromuscular junction with decreased acetylcholine effect	Anticholinesterases Steroids Thymectomy Plasmapheresis
Myasthenic syndrome (Eaton-Lambert)	Middle-aged M	Gradual onset of proximal weakness associated with carcinoma (oat cell) of lung	Proximal muscle weakness with atrophy Respiratory distress	EMG-incremental response on high frequency (greater than 10 cycles/second) stimulation	Decreased acetylcholine release at neuromuscular junction	Remove underlying malignancy Guanidine (35 mg/kg/day) through nasogastric tube (increases release of acetylcholine at neuromuscular junction) Steroids Plasmapheresis
Landry-Guillain-Barré syndrome	Any age or sex	Subacute onset of peripheral numbness with progressive (distal to proximal) weakness, usually after flu-like disease or inoculation	Dysesthesias Facial paralysis Global weakness Absent DTRs Respiratory failure	CSF-increased protein with small cellular response (albumino-cytologic dissociation) Nerve conduction velocities slowed Elevation of Epstein-Barr virus antibody titer	Immune response to virus affecting nerves, roots, and possibly root entry zone at spinal cord level	
Botulism	Any age or sex	Generalized paralysis Bulbar symptoms Respiratory failure	Dysarthria Ophthalmoplegia Dysphagia Autonomic changes Decreased DTRs	EMG may mimic myasthenic syndrome Mouse inoculation test for presence of toxin Stool culture	Botulinis toxin inhibits acetylcholine release at neuromuscular junction	Appropriate antitoxin to botulinis toxin (ABE forms) Guanidine
Poliomyelitis	Any age or sex	Fever, nuchal rigidity Diffuse muscle pain Bulbar symptoms Focal weakness	Focal asymmetric weakness Decreased DTRs Respiratory depression Bulbar findings Muscle pain Meningeal signs	EMG focal denervation CSF increased protein with increased cellular response (polymorphonuclear leukocytes early, lymphocytes late) Increased antibody titer to poliovirus	An acute infection with poliovirus that attacks the anterior horn cell	Vaccination and prevention Supportive and symptomatic management Physiatric and orthopedic rehabilitation

TABLE 13–13.
Neuromuscular Diseases Characteristically Displaying Facial Alterations*

FACIAL COMPONENT	ALTERATION	CHARACTERISTIC DISEASE
Eyes	Ptosis	Myasthenia gravis
		Ocular myopathy
		Oculopharyngeal myopathy
		Dystrophia myotonica
	Ophthalmoplegia	Ocular myopathy
		Oculo-cranio-somatic neuromuscular disease
		Oculopharyngeal myopathy
	Bell's sign	Facioscapulohumeral dystrophy
Mouth	Lip protrusion	Facioscapulohumeral dystrophy
	Triangular lips	Neonatal dystrophia myotonica
		Praeder-Willi syndrome
	Tapir-like	Dystrophia myotonica
	Macroglossia with orthodontic pathology	Duchenne muscular dystrophy
Skin	Butterfly rash	Dermatomyositis
	Heliotrope rash	
	Periorbital edema	
	Flattening of nasolabial folds and other loss of facial lines	Facioscapulohumeral dystrophy
	Fasciculations	Spinal muscular atrophy
		Amyotrophic lateral sclerosis
		Dystrophia myotonica
Hair	Temporal balding	Myasthenia gravis
Jaw	Masseter weakness/wasting	Oculopharyngeal myopathy
		Dystrophia myotonica
	Masseter hypertrophy	Duchenne muscular dystrophy
Total Facial Countenance	Mask-like	Facioscapulohumeral dystrophy
	Dysmorphic (long, thin)	Morphologically specific myopathies
	Lugubrious	Dystrophia myotonica
	Diplegia	Neonatal dystrophia myotonica
		Mobius syndrome
	"Snarling" smile	Myasthenia gravis

*From Siegel I: The many faces of neuromuscular disease. *Postgrad Med* 1986; 7:121–137. Used by permission.

BIBLIOGRAPHY

Appel SH: The muscular dystrophies: Clinical update on two major types. *Postgrad Med* 1978; 64:93–102.

Askari A, Vignos PJ, Moskowitz RW: Steroid myopathy in connective tissue disease. *Am J Med* 1976; 61:485–492.

Becker KL: Corticosteroids: Many of their side effects are really their actions. *Drug Therapy/Hospital* 1981; December, pp 75–80.

Bethlem J: *Myopathies.* Philadelphia, JB Lippincott, Co, 1977.

Bohan A, Peter JB: Polymyositis and dermatomyositis (Part 1). *N Engl J Med* 1975; 292:344–349.

Bohan A, Peter JB: Polymyositis and dermatomyositis (Part 2). *N Engl J Med* 1975; 292:403–407.

Bonsett CA: Prophylactic bracing in pseudohypertrophic muscular dystrophy (preliminary report) *Indiana Med* 1975; 68:181–187.

Boshes LD: Diseases of muscles, clinical manifestations, and differential diagnosis. *New Physician* 1967; 16:263–274.

Brain L, Walton JN: *Brain's Diseases of the Nervous System,* ed 7. London, Oxford University Press, 1969.

Brooke MH: Muscular dystrophies and congenital myopathies. *Neurol Neurosurg* 1979; 36:2–7.

Caughey JE, Myrianthopoulos NC: Dystrophia myotonica and related disorders. Springfield, Illinois, Charles C Thomas, Publisher, 1963.

Chhabra SL: Roussy-Levy syndrome and Charcot-Marie-Tooth disease. *Orthop Rev* 1983; 2:65–69.

Chyatte SB, Rudman D, Patterson JH, et al: Human growth hormone and estrogens in boys with Duchenne muscular dystrophy. *Arch Phys Med Rehabil* 1973; 54:248–253.

Croft P: Carcinomatous neuromyopathy. *Practitioner* 1976; April, pp 407–413.

Dau PC: Plasmapheresis in idiopathic inflammatory myopathy. *Arch Neurol* 1981; 38:544–560.

Dickey RP, Ziter FA, Smith RA: Emery-Dreifuss muscular dystrophy. *J Pediatr* 1984; 104:555–559.

Dowben RM: Prolonged survival of dystrophic mice treated with 17-Ethyl-19 nortestosterone. *Nature* 1959; 184:1966–1967.

Drachman DA: Ophthalmoplegia plus, The neurodegenerative disorders associated with progressive external ophthalmoplegia. *Arch Neurol* 1968; 18:654–674.

Dubowitz V: The floppy infant, in *Clinics in Developmental Medicine,* No 31. London, William Heinemann Medical Books Ltd, (Spastics International Medical Publications), 1969.

Dubowitz V: *Muscle Disorders in Childhood.* Philadelphia, WB Saunders Co, 1978.

Duchenne de Boulogne GBA: Recherches sur la paralysie musculaire pseudohypertrophique, ou paralysie myosclerosique. *Archives Generales de Medecine* 1868; (6 ser): 11.

Dujovne CA, Azarnoff DL: Clinical complications of corticosteroid therapy: A selected review. *Med Clin North Am* 1973; 57:1331–1342.

Dyken PR, Harper PS: Congenital dystrophia myotonica. *Neurology* (Minneapolis) 1973; 23:465–473.

Engel WK: Myotonia: A different point of view. *Calif Med* 1971; 114:32–37.

Enomoto A, Bradley WG: Therapeutic trials in muscular dystrophy. *Arch Neurol* 1977; 34:771–773.

Evans FA, Drennan JC, Russman BS: Functional classification and orthopaedic management of spinal muscular atrophy. *J Bone Joint Surg (Br)* 1981; 4:516–522.

Ford FF: *Diseases of the Nervous System in Infancy, Childhood, and Adolescence*, ed 5. Springfield, Illinois, Charles C Thomas, Publisher, 1966.

Fowler WM, Jr: Rehabilitation management of muscular dystrophy and related disorders: II. Comprehensive care. *Arch Phys Med Rehabil* 1982; 63:322–328.

Fredericks EJ, Russman BS: Bedside evaluation of large motor units in childhood spinal muscular atrophy. *Neurology* 1979; 29:398–400.

Galdi AP: *Diagnosis and Management of Muscle Disease*. New York, SP Medical & Scientific Books, 1984.

Girdany B, Danowski TS: Muscular dystrophy. *Am J Dis Child* 1956; 91:339–345.

Goebel HH, Muller J, DeMyer W: Myopathy associated with Marfan's syndrome. *Neurology* (Minneapolis) 1973; 23:1257–1268.

Greene RD (ed): *Myasthenia Gravis*. Philadelphia, JB Lippincott, Co, 1969.

Gucker T, III: Sorting out the muscle diseases. Consultant. 1971; 4:19–21.

Haas DC: Treatment of polymyositis with immunosuppressive drugs. *Neurology* 1973; 23:55–62.

Haleem MA: Myopathies in the elderly. *Gerontologia Clinica* 1972; 14:361–377.

Harper P: *Myotonic Dystrophy*. Philadelphia, WB Saunders Co, 1979.

Harter JG, Reddy WJ, Thorn GW: Studies on an intermittent corticosteroid dosage regimen. *N Engl J Med* 1963; 269:591–596.

Hughes JT, Brownell B: Pathology of peroneal muscular atrophy (Charcot-Marie-Tooth disease). *J Neurol Neurosurg Psychiatry* 1972; 35:648–657.

Jackson CE, Strehler DA: Limb-girdle muscular dystrophy: Clinical manifestations and detection of preclinical disease. *Pediatrics* 1968; 41:495–502.

Kamoshita S, Konishi Y, Segawa M, et al: Congenital muscular dystrophy as a disease of the central nervous system. *Arch Neurol* 1976; 33:513–516.

Kaneda RR: Becker's muscular dystrophy: Orthopedic implications. *J Am Osteopath Assoc* 1980; 79:332–335.

Kaplan PE: Rheumatoid myopathy. IMJ 1977; February, pp 106–110.

Khan RH, MacNicol MF: Bilateral patellar subluxation secondary to Becker muscular dystrophy (A case report). *J Bone Joint Surg (Am)* 1982; 5:77–78.

Larsen WG: Polymyositis dermatomyositis. *Arch Dermatol* 1967; 96:724–727.

Ludman H: Dysphagia in dystrophia myotonica. *J Laryngol Otol* 1962; 76:234–236.

McComas AJ, Upton ARM, Sica REP: Motoneurone disease and aging. *Lancet* 1973; 29:1477–1480.

McComas AJ, Sica REP, Upton ARM: Multiple muscle analysis of motor units in muscular dystrophy. *Arch Neurol* 1974; 30:249–251.

Malpe RR, Lee MHM, Alba A (eds): Rehabilitation technics in polymyositis. *NY State J Med* 1973; 73:1208–1210.

Margolis MD, Freitas WJ, Margolis LS: Hypothyroidism mimicking myotonic dystrophy. *J Am Geriatr Soc* 1973; 21:31–32.

Mulder D (ed): *The Diagnosis and Treatment of Amyotrophic Lateral Sclerosis.* Boston, Houghton Mifflin Co, 1980.

Nelson TE, Flewellen EH: Current concepts: The malignant hyperthermia syndrome. *N Engl J Med* 1983; 309:416–418.

Ogg E: Milestones in muscle disease research. Muscular Dystrophy Association of America, Inc, 1971.

Olson ND, Jou MF, Quast JE, et al: Peripheral neuropathy in myotonic dystrophy. *Arch Neurol* 1978; 35:741–746.

Olson W, Engel WK, Walsh GO, et al: Oculocraniosomatic neuromuscular disease with "ragged-red" fibers. *Arch Neurol* 1972; 26:193–210.

Panayiotopoulos CP, Scarpalezos S: Hypertrophy of extensor digitorum brevis in limb-girdle muscular dystrophy. *Lancet* 1974; ii:230.

Patel AN, Kumara SR: Muscle percussion and neostigmine test in the clinical evaluation of neuromuscular disorders. *N Engl J Med* 1969; 281:523–526.

Pearn JH, Wilson J: Acute Werdnig-Hoffmann disease, acute infantile spinal muscular atrophy. *Arch Dis Child* 1973; 48:425–430.

Pearson CM: Muscular dystrophy (review and recent observations). *Am J Med* 1963; 35:632–645.

Perlstein MA: Deep-tendon reflexes in pseudohypertrophic muscular dystrophy, rate and order of loss. *JAMA* 1965; 193:540–541.

Polgar JG, Bradley WG, Upton ARM, et al: The early detection of dystrophia myotonica. *Brain* 1972; 95:761–776.

Pruzanski W, Huvos AG: Smooth muscle involvement in primary muscle disease. I. Myotonic dystrophy. *Arch Pathol* 1967; 83:229–233.

Reinherz R, Mann I: Lower extremity involvement in Duchenne's muscular dystrophy. *J Am Podiatr Med Assoc* 1977; 67:796–801.

Rennie MJ, Edwards RHT, Millward DJ, et al: Effects of Duchenne muscular dystrophy on muscle protein synthesis. *Nature* 1982; 296:165–167.

Review of Current Concepts of Myopathies: Clinical Orthopaedics and Related Research, no 39. Philadelphia, JB Lippincott, Co, 1965.

Rosen AD: Amyotrophic lateral sclerosis: Clinical features and prognosis. *Arch Neurol* 1978; 35:638–642.

Rowland LP, Fetell M, Olarte M, et al: Emery-Dreifuss muscular dystrophy. *Ann Neurol* 1979; 5:111–117.

Russman BS, Melchreit R, Drennan JC: Spinal muscular atrophy: The natural course of disease. *Muscle Nerve* 1983; 6:179–181.

Scarpalezos S, Panayiotopoulos CP: Duchenne muscular dystrophy: Reservations to the neurogenic hypothesis. *Lancet* 1973; ii:458.

Schott GD, Wills MR: Muscle weakness in osteomalacia. *Lancet* 1976; Mar 20:626–629.

Seybold ME: Myasthenia gravis. *JAMA* 1983; 250:2516–2521.

Shy GM: The late onset myopathy. *World Neurol* 1962; 3:149–160.

Siegel IM: Early signs of Landouzy-Dejerine disease: Wrist and finger weakness. JAMA (letter) 1972; 221:302.

Siegel IM: Very early diagnosis of Duchenne muscular dystrophy. *Lancet* 1976; 2:90.

Siegel IM: Foot deformity in myotubular myopathy: Pathology of intrinsic foot musculature. *Arch Neurol* 1983; 40:589.

Sinaki M, Mulder DW: Rehabilitation techniques for patients with amyotrophic lateral sclerosis. *Mayo Clin Proc* 1978; 53:173–178.

Skouteli H, Dubowitz V: Fasciculation of the eyelids: An additional clue to clinical diagnosis in spinal muscular atrophy. *Neuropediatrics* 1984; 15:145–146.

Smith R, Stern G: Muscular weakness in osteomalacia and hyperparathyroidism. *J Neurol Sci* 1969; 8:511–520.

Smith RA, Norris FH, Jr: Symptomatic care of patients with amyotrophic lateral sclerosis. *JAMA* 1975; 234:715–717.

Swash M, Schwartz M: Neuromuscular diseases. New York, Springer-Verlag, 1981.

Takahashi K, Oimomi M, Shinko T, et al: Response of serum creatine phosphokinase to steroid hormone. *Arch Neurol* 1975; 32:89–92.

Tyler JH, Sutherland JM: The primary spinocerebellar atrophies and their associated defects, with a study of the foot deformity. *Brain* 1961; 84:289–300.

Van Der Meulen JP: Acute weakness. *Emerg Med* 1984; Oct 30:80–106.

Van Wijngaarden GK, Bethlem J: Benign infantile spinal muscular atrophy: A prospective study. Brain 1973; 96:163–170.

Vick NA: Disease of skeletal muscle: Current ideas of diagnosis and management. *Chicago Med* 1973; 76:621–625.

Walton JN: (ed): *Disorders of Voluntary Muscles,* ed 4. New York, Churchill Livingstone, Inc, 1981.

Wilner EC, Brody JA: An evolution of the remote effects of lung cancer on the central nervous system. *Neurology* (Minneapolis) 1968; 18:287.

Winkelman RK, Mulder DW, Lambert EH, et al: Course of dermatomyositis-polymyositis: Comparison of untreated and cortisone-treated patients. *Mayo Clin Proc* 1968; 43:546–556.

Young RSK, Gang DL, Zalneraitis EL, et al: Dysmaturation in infants of mothers with myotonic dystrophy. *Arch Neurol* 1981; 38:716–719.

Zundel WS, Tyler FH: The muscular dystrophies (Birth defects reprint series). *N Engl J Med* 1965; 273:537–543, 596–601.

PART IV

Management of Neuromuscular Diseases

14

Muscle Weakness

"Care more particularly for the individual patient than for the special features of the disease."

Sir William Osler (1849–1919)

The cause and cure of most muscle disease is unknown. Incurable, however, is not synonymous with untreatable. Many supportive and symptomatic aids are available and, through proper therapy, comfort, functional capacity, and even life expectancy can be significantly increased.

Although remarks concerning treatment are found at appropriate points throughout the text, this section is devoted entirely to such measures. Though specific therapy for a variety of neuromuscular conditions is covered, Duchenne muscular dystrophy, because of its rapidly progressive course and ultimate severe disability, is used as a model for analysis of those force imbalances that shape skeletal deformity. Comments concerning pathokinetic mechanisms as well as orthopedic management can, to a large degree, be applied appropriately to any of the other muscular dystrophies.

DISTRIBUTION OF MUSCLE WEAKNESS

I. The muscle formed first in the embryo, axial musculature, and that of the limb girdles is initially and most severely involved in DMD.

175

Most major axial or appendicular musculature requires at least 30%–40% anatomic loss before clinical weakness becomes obvious.

A. This accounts for apparent normal functioning of children with DMD during the first years of life.

B. The abiotrophic half-life of muscle in DMD is 4.8 years.

C. Improvement in some patients from 5–7 years of age can be explained by the processes of normal development outstripping progression of the disease during this period.

D. The mechanical efficiency of the skeleton probably doubles as the body matures.
   1. Skeletal mass increases 20 times from the newborn to the adult.
   2. Muscle mass increases 40 times.

E. A greater proportion of muscle is required as the limbs grow, since work necessary to move an appendage is proportional to the fourth power of its length, whereas that achieved by muscle is proportional to the cube of its length.
   1. The scale effect (first described by Galileo) tells us that for every unit linear increase in a solid body, the surface area of the body increases by the square of the unit, its volume by the unit cubed (Fig 14–1).
      a) This explains why a patient with even an inactive condition limiting his ultimate muscle mass may, although initially ambulatory, eventually lose the ability to walk with growth.

II. From a rehabilitation standpoint, the sum of muscle weakness, contracture, and imbalance determines a patient's ability to perform (Fig 14–2). The muscle regression curve in DMD indicates that below age 7.5 years, there is little or no functional change in 75% of patients over a single year. Beyond age 7.5 years, 75% of patients show significant functional change each year.

A. Standard muscle testing is not sensitive enough to evaluate the functional status of muscle groups, depending as they do on a delicate agonist-antagonist balance.

B. Muscle activity is a complex operation depending upon a prime mover working in concert with antagonists, synergists and stabilizers.

C. Also of importance are the relative activities of those muscles stabilizing position (tonic) and those that mostly activate movement (phasic).
   1. Spurt muscles, such as the biceps brachii, tend to atrophy earlier in myopathy than shunt muscles, such as the brachioradialis.

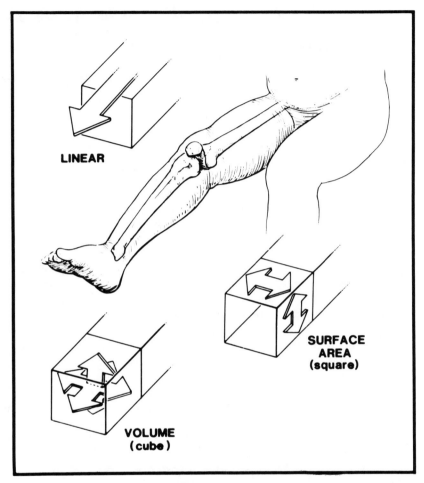

FIG 14–1.
The scale effect.

2. The gastroc-soleus muscle combination is the most powerful in the body. Its strength is four times as great as the maximal isometric tension its muscles can develop; it supports a force almost three times body weight through the toe-heel lever arm during walking take-off.

D. Any change in range of motion of a joint against gravity is interpreted as indicating a change in muscular strength. Some muscles perform certain functions at specific positions of joint or body segment angulation. For instance, whereas semimem-

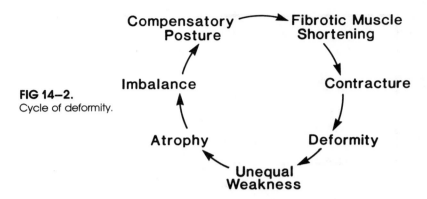

FIG 14–2.
Cycle of deformity.

branosus, semitendinosus, biceps femoris, gluteus maximus, and middle and inferior portions of adductor magnus can produce hip extension at any angle of pelvifemoral extension, gracilis and superior portion of adductor magnus become extensors between 165 and 150 degrees, adductor brevis between 135 and 150 degrees, and adductor longus near 120 degrees of extension of the pelvis on the femora. It is common experience that one can exert greater grip strength in the preferred functional position (30 degrees wrist extension). Tension is decreased with hyperflexion or hyperextension of the wrist because the optimal fiber length for this task is at 30 degrees of wrist extension. Similarly, more energy (37%) is required to function with a knee restricted at 135 degrees extension (20% more with a knee stiff in full extension) or a hip (13% more) at 180 degrees.

1. Muscle imbalance is as important a factor as specific muscle weakness in compromising motor function.
2. Malalignment of weight-bearing joints can aggravate the effect of muscle weakness on ambulation.
3. Muscles shortened by contracture develop less maximal tension than they could otherwise. They also fatigue more rapidly.

PHYSICAL THERAPY

I. The roles that the physical therapist plays in the management of the patient with muscular dystrophy are several.
   A. The therapist monitors the assessment of specific muscle weaknesses, imbalance, and contracture (Table 14–1).

TABLE 14–1.
Assessment

Strength and range of motion: shoulders, hips, knees.
Contractures: hip flexors, tensor fasciae, and heel cords.
Function: rising, stairs, walking, etc.

1. Muscle testing grades key muscles as to strength and range of motion of activated joints against gravity (Fig 14–3). Computerized dynamometers are now available for such testing.
2. The patient's ability to perform a number of standard tasks is assessed, measuring time required and observing method employed to complete the task (Fig 14–4). Subtle alterations in method as well as slight changes in time needed for any given task objectively reflect changes in strength.
3. The patient can be rated on a functional 10-step scale.
   a) Stage 1, walks and climbs stairs without assistance (it takes 15 times as much energy to ascend a flight of ordinary stairs as to walk a level distance equal to the vertical height of the stairs).
   b) Stage 2, walks and climbs stairs easily with aid of railing.
   c) Stage 3, walks and climbs stairs slowly with aid of railing.
   d) Stage 4, walks but cannot climb stairs.
   e) Stage 5, walks unassisted but cannot climb stairs or get out of chair.
   f) Stage 6, walks only with assistance or with braces.
   g) Stage 7, in wheelchair, sits erect and can roll chair and perform bed and wheelchair activities of daily living.
   h) Stage 8, in wheelchair, sits erect but is unable to perform bed and chair activities without assistance.
   i) Stage 9, in wheelchair, sits erect only with support, and able to do only minimal activities of daily living.
   j) Stage 10, in bed, cannot perform activities of daily living without assistance.
4. The kinetic sequence of the above scale provides a treatment format for the physical therapy program.
   a) In stages 1–3, the patient is ambulating independently. Passive stretch of early lower extremity contractures may be necessary by stage 3. Functional activities of daily living and ambulation are sufficient active exercise for stages 1–3.
   b) Between stages 5–6, lower extremity surgery is indicated because contracture leads to increased difficulty with anti-

Left   *Right*

					DATE				
					THERAPIST				
					Neck flexors				
					Abdominals				
					Scapular winging				
					Shoulder abduction				
					Shoulder extension				
					Elbow flexion				
					Elbow extension				
					Wrist extension				
					Hip extension				
					Hip abduction				
					Hip flexion				
					Knee extension				
					Knee flexion				
					Foot dorsiflexion				
					Foot plantar flexion				
					Foot eversion				
					Foot inversion				
					Pseudohypertrophy measurement*				

*Circumference at widest part of calf.

Left   *Right*

					CONTRACTURES				
					Hip				
					TFL				
					Knee				
					Ankle				
					Elbow				
					Lag				
					Hip				
					Knee				
					Total				

Explanation of Testing Procedures Modified Muscle Testing

Anterior Neck Musculature

Patient is supine on table. Flexes neck. Resist on forehead and grade *normal* to *fair*. If patient does not have ability to flex antigravity, test sidelying and grade *poor* to *zero*.

Abdominal Musculature

Patient is supine on table with knees flexed and feet held by therapist. He attempts to sit up with hands behind head for normal grade (four to five full sit-ups), arms folded across chest for good, arms extended at sides for fair. If patient is unable to do full sit-up in fair position, measure in inches the distance he is able to lift the seventh cervical vertebra from surface and palpate abdominal muscles.

Note: If anterior neck musculature is poor, support head to test for abdominal strength.

FIG 14–3.
Modified muscle testing and goniometry.

Scapular Winging
The patient is sitting and an attempt is made to lift patient at both axillas. If the patient 'slips through' and the scapulae become more prominent, it indicates a weakness of the serratus anterior and other shoulder girdle musculature. This should be marked 'yes' or 'no' on the form.

Shoulder Abduction
Patient sits straight with arms at sides, then, with palms down, raises arms to sides and over head bilaterally to avoid substitution. Do not allow patient to come into flexion. If patient has full range of motion, resist at elbows to 90° abduction and grade *normal* to *fair*. If patient has less than full antigravity range of motion, measure the degree of motion with the goniometer axis at the shoulder joint, using a line parallel to the midline of the body for one arm, the midline of the humerus for the other.
If patient has no antigravity motion, test in the supine position and grade from *poor* to *zero*.

Shoulder Extension
Patient is prone on table, arm over edge and shoulder flexed to 90°. Extends shoulder with palm up while scapula is stabilized. If patient has full range of antigravity motion, measure the angle, calling 90° of shoulder flexion (starting position 0° extension) and measuring up toward full extension (approximately 125°) down the midline of the humerus toward lateral epicondyle with axis at the shoulder joint. Give assistance at elbow at neutral position (90° extension from starting position) and grade *normal* to *fair*. If patient has less than full range of antigravity motion, measure angle of extension as described above. Resist as able. If patient has no antigravity extension, measure sidelying and grade *poor* to *zero*.

Elbow Flexion
Patient sits with arms at sides, elbows fully extended, then flexes one elbow; may use all elbow flexors. If patient has full range of motion, give resistance at wrist and grade *normal* to *fair*. If patient lacks full range against gravity, elbow may be set in initial flexion to achieve full range; this is then noted. If patient has no antigravity flexion, position supine and attempt elbow flexion, grading *poor* to *zero*.

Elbow Extension
Patient is prone on table, arm over edge and shoulder flexed to 90°. Extends shoulder with palm up while scapula is stabilized. If patient has full range of antigravity motion, give resistance at wrist and grade *normal* to *fair*. If patient has less than full range, measure from 90° flexion to degree of extensor lag using lateral epicondyle as axis and aligning one arm with greater tubercle of humerus, the other with radial head and record 90 to degree of lag as active motion (example 90–20°). If patient has no antigravity extension, position supine and grade *poor* to *zero*.

Wrist Extension
Patient sits with elbow flexed to 90°, extends wrist with fingers relaxed. If patient has full range of motion, antigravity, give resistance to extension and grade *normal* to *fair*. If patient has less than full antigravity motion, grade fair minus. If patient lacks antigravity motion, attempt extension with hand supported on ulnar border and grade *poor* to *zero*.

Hip Extension
Patient is prone over edge of table with trunk supported, hips flexed to 90°, knees extended and feet on floor. Keeping knee straight, patient extends hip through range. If patient has full range of antigravity motion, resist at knee and grade *normal* to *fair*. If patient has less than full range, measure the degree of hip extension from 90° flexion through range, using greater trochanter as axis and the midline of the trunk and lateral

FIG 14–3. *(cont.)* *(continued)*

condyle of femur as sights for the goniometer arms. Record (example, 90–30°, 60° active motion). Resist as able. If patient has no antigravity hip extension, position sidelying and grade *poor* to *zero*.

Note: If patient has full range of motion, may also test prone on the table and extend hip with knee extended and grade *normal* to *fair*.

Hip Abduction

Patient is in the sidelying position with the leg slightly extended beyond the midline. The patient abducts the leg through range of motion for fair grade; resist at the knee for good to normal. Poor grade is tested in supine position.

Hip Flexion

The patient is sitting with both knees flexed to 90°. Patient flexes one hip through range of motion for fair grade; resist at the knee for good to normal. Poor grade muscle is tested in sidelying position with upper leg supported, patient flexes hip through range of motion.

Knee Extension

Patient sits with hip and knee flexed to 90°, hands in lap. Extends knee through range of motion while maintaining erect posture. If patient has full range, give resistance at ankle and grade *normal* to *fair*. If patient lacks full range, measure from 90° flexion to limit of extension using lateral condyle of femur as axis with one arm of goniometer aligned with greater trochanter, the other with lateral malleolus. Record extensor lag and degree of motion (example 90–30°, 60° active motion). Resist as able and grade. If patient has no antigravity extension, test in sidelying and grade *poor* to *zero*.

Knee Flexion

The patient is supine and flexes knee through range of motion for fair grade. Resist for good to normal. Poor grade is tested with patient sidelying and upper leg supported, patient flexes knee.

Foot Dorsiflexion

Patient is supine on table. From position of plantar flexion, he dorsiflexes and resistance is given on dorsal aspect of foot; grade *normal* to *fair*. If patient lacks full range, grade fair minus. If patient has no antigravity dorsiflexion, position sidelying and grade *poor* to *zero*.

Foot Plantar Flexion

Tested with patient standing and being albe to stand on toes of the foot for good to normal grade. Fair grade is tested with patient prone and foot extended over edge of table at 90°, patient plantar flexes foot.

Foot Eversion

Tested with patient supine. Patient everts foot from plantar flexed position. Resist at lateral border of foot for good to normal grade. Tested sidelying for fair grade, and patient everts foot through range of motion.

Foot Inversion

Tested in supine position. Patient inverts foot through range of motion for fair grade; resist at medial border of forefoot for good to normal grades.

Measurement of Contractures

Hip flexion Contracture

Measure in Thomas position, one knee flexed to chest, allowing no lordosis, extend other leg avoiding any abduction. Measure along midline of trunk and toward lateral femoral condyle with axis of goniometer at greater trochanter.

FIG 14–3. *(cont.)*

Tensor Fascia Lata Tightness
Measure prone with leg abducted to eliminate as much hip flexion contracture as possible and cause maximum relaxation of tensor. Flex knee to 90°, exert pressure on sacrum and adduct leg until hip flexes further. Measure angle of abduction with one arm of goniometer on posterior iliac spines, other arm extending down midline of posterior aspect of leg.

Knee Flexion Contracture
Measure with patient supine, legs extended to greatest degree possible, using lateral femoral condyle as axis and sighting to greater trochanter and lateral malleolus.

Plantar Flexion Contracture
Measure in test position for foot dorsiflexion. Exert pressure on plantar surface of foot to insure maximum passive dorsiflexion. Measure laterally along fibula and plantar surface of foot. Record dorsiflexion of plantar flexion contracture.

Elbow Flexion Contracture
Measure in test position for elbow extension, assist to full passive extension when necessary. Place arms of goniometer along midline of humerus and radius as described under testing procedures for elbow extension.

FIG 14–3. *(concluded)*

gravity activities. Where contracture is minimal or absent, orthotic modifications or bracing alone may be sufficient to augment weakened knee extension and keep the patient ambulating. With fair quadriceps strength, the knee flexion moment can be decreased by an anteriorly placed cushioned (SACH type) heel, or converted to an extension moment with an equinus (floor reaction) AFO (Fig 14–5).

  c) Ambulant patients in stages 5 and 6 should not avoid activity and use wheelchairs, except when absolutely necessary and then for only brief periods of time.

  d) Stage 7 should not be skipped as the patient is thus condemned to stage 10 immediately.

  e) When stage 7 is reached, routine conditioning exercises are prescribed to retard disuse atrophy and maintain independence in wheelchair activities. Prophylactic treatment of scoliosis is also initiated at this time as well as a full program of respiratory therapy.

  f) Obesity is usually a problem after stage 6.

  g) The closer a patient is to stage 10, the more assistive devices he requires.

B. The therapist instructs and supervises patients in exercises, stretching, and gait training, directed toward improving muscular strength as well as preventing and correcting contracture, thus increasing efficiency in the functional activities of daily living, including TDL and transfer.

Name:													
Activity	Date Therapist												
1. Run 25 feet					Time to Accomplish Task								
2. Walk 25 feet	a. Independent												
	b. Short leg braces												
	c. Long leg braces												
	d. Crutches, walker or cane												
3. Climb 8 stairs	a. Independent—foot over foot												
	b. Independent—one step at a time												
	c. Hands on knees												
	d. Railing—one hand												
	e. Railing and hand on knee												
	f. Railing—two hands												
4. Walk down 8 stairs	a. Independent												
	b. Railing—one hand												
	c. Railing—two hands												
5. Rise from chair	a. Independent												
	b. Gower's sign												
	c. Turn to side, then push up												
	d. Pull up with aid of table												
6. Role over from supine to prone													
7. Roll over from prone to supine													
8. Get to all-fours position from prone													
9. Sit up from Supine	a. Independent												
	b. Pull up												
	c. Pull up and push on elbows												
	d. Turn to side, then push up												
	e. To hand and knees, then sit up												
10. Rise from floor from prone position	a. Independent												
	b. Gower's sign												
	c. Chair to standing												
	d. Chair to sitting, then to standing												
11. Sitting balance	a. Stable												
	b. Unstable												
12. Vital capacity—sitting													
13. Height													
14. Weight													
15. Hand grip	a. Right												
	b. Left												

EXPLANATION OF TESTING PROCEDURES
FUNCTIONAL ASSESSMENT CHART
ACTIVITY—timed (1 through 10) and observed (11)

1. **Run 25 feet**
   Both feet off the ground at one time.

FIG 14—4.
Functional assessment chart.

2. Walk 25 feet
  a. Independent—no assistance from mechanical aids.
  b. Short leg braces—test items 3, 4, and 5 with braces also.
  c. Long leg braces—test items, 3, 4, and 5 with braces also.
  d. Crutches, walker or cane.
     Stair measurements: Depth—11½"; height—7"; railing height—36".

3. Climb 8 stairs
  a. Independent—foot over foot—no assistance such as pushing on knee, using rail.
  b. Independent—one step at a time.
  c. Hands on knees—assistance from rail.
  d. Railing—one hand.
  e. Railing and hand on knee—patient pulls on rail with one hand, pushes on knee with the other.
  f. Railing—two hands, some patients may use two rails

4. Walk down 8 stairs
  a. Independent—no assistance from rail. May go foot over foot, or one step at a time.
  b. Railing—one hand, often used for safety but not for support.
  c. Railing—two hands, or rail and therapist's hand for safety.

5. Rise from chair
Care must be taken to seat the patient in a chair which places his feet flat on the floor and his knees in 90° flexion. This is particularly important with children as a higher chair would give them a mechanical advantage.

  a. Independent—rising without pushing on chair or knees, arms folded across chest or extended.
  b. Gower's sign—includes pressure on knees or pressure on seat of chair or both.
  c. Turn to side, then push up—patient turns sideways in chair to sit on one hip, with feet on floor pushes with arms to 90° hip flexion and pushes off to upright position or climbs up chair to upright position.
  d. Pull up with aid of table—patient takes support from table with hips flexed while extending knees. Once knees are locked, patient extends hips by pushing up on table.

6. Roll over from supine to prone
Contractures may inhibit this activity.

7. Roll over from prone to supine
Contractures may inhibit this activity.

8. Get to all-fours position from prone
Push up to hands and knees.

9. Sit up from supine
  a. independent—no aids other than having ankles held down by therapist which is within the range of normal; must achieve sitting balance.
  b. pull up—patient holds on to leg or clothing to pull himself up.
  c. pull and push on elbow—begins to pull up, then pushes on at least one elbow.
  d. turn to side, then push up—patient will roll to side, then push up with both arms to achieve sitting balance.
  e. to hands and knees, then sit up—roll to prone, to hands and knees, then to side sit or other sitting balance.

10. Rise from floor from prone position
  a. Independent—no assistance required.
  b. Gower's sign—can bring himself to his feet but must push on knees to assume erect posture.

FIG 14—4. *(cont.)*   *(continued)*

    c. Chair to standing—patient pulls himself to feet with aid of chair, then pushes on chair to achieve upright position.

    d. Chair to sitting, then to standing—patient pulls himself to sitting position in chair, then pushes himself to upright position, using chair.

    Patient should be placed on edge of table with thighs fully supported and knees flexed to 90°.

11. Sitting balance
  a. Stable
  b. Unstable—patient sits erect but cannot recover balance if it is lost. Or, patient is unable to maintain his balance without support of his arms.

12. Vital capacity
Measured sitting, taking highest of two readings. Take height and weight into consideration.

13. Height.

14. Weight.

15. Hand grip
Measured with Newman myometer taking highest of two readings for left and right hands. Keep arms at side during measurement.

FIG 14–4. *(concluded)*

1. Overenthusiastic stretching of contractures should be avoided because it produces pain and stimulates the stretch reflex, strengthening deforming muscles by prompting the patient to fight the passive force by an active effort of his own.

2. Disability from weakness must be distinguished from that caused by contracture. The essential tenodesis effect of contracture (secondary to changes in muscle length-tension relationship) in the face of severe loss of muscular support should be monitored by the therapist. Initially such compen-

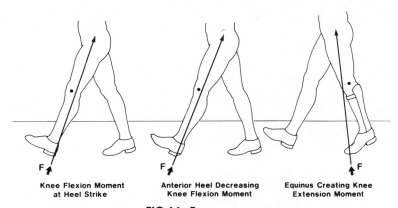

| Knee Flexion Moment at Heel Strike | Anterior Heel Decreasing Knee Flexion Moment | Equinus Creating Knee Extension Moment |

FIG 14–5.
Ground force reaction.

sating mechanisms help maintain proper body alignment. Eventually they contribute to ambulatory loss.

3. Muscular activity enhances contractile protein synthesis.
   a) At complete rest, strength is lost at a rate of approximately 3% to 5% a day. *("What we don't use, we lose.")*
   b) Endurance (which depends also on cardiovascular capacity) is also limited.
   c) The maximal daily tension exerted must be greater than 20% of maximal muscular strength or strength will decrease.
      (1) For improved performance, overload is required.
      (2) Endurance training is required to increase the oxidative capacity of muscle.
4. Three processes contribute to the deformities of muscular dystrophy.
   a) Muscle weakness.
   b) Muscle imbalance.
   c) Specific muscle contractures secondary to gravity and compensatory postural habitus. Often contracture is asymmetrical and less in dominant limbs because of relative increased activity.
5. It is desirable to maintain physical function though an aggressive program of physical therapy that provides:
   a) Maximal isotonic resistance or submaximal isokinetic resistance exercises.
      (1) DMD, LGD, and FSH have demonstrated definite but limited increase in muscle strength with exercise, but heavy exercise may potentially accelerate weakness, leading to metabolic bankruptcy.
      (2) Potential for increasing muscle strength is related to the preexercise strength of the muscle.
      (3) For maximal salutary effect, exercise programs in DMD should be initiated early in the course of the disease.
   b) Gait training and pivot transfer.
   c) Contracture stretching (particularly hip flexors, tensor fasciae latae, and heel cords) (Table 14–2).
6. Nonexhausting functional exercises may be helpful in maintaining strength.
7. Passive stretching of contractures can, by balancing agonist against antagonist, prolong function and decrease the energy cost of muscular activity to the patient.
8. Proper physical therapy should preserve the balance neces-

TABLE 14–2.
Exercises for Stretching Key Musculature

MUSCLES	ACTIVE	PASSIVE
Hip flexors	Lying supine at edge of bed or table, hold opposite knee and hip flexed, drop leg over edge and allow weight of extremity to extend hip.	Patient prone—knees extended—while stabilizing hip from behind elevate knee from the table.
Tensor fascia (iliotibial band)	Stand with one side toward wall and feet about 8–12 inches from the wall. Keep knees straight and lean the near hip toward the wall.	Patient prone, thigh extended and abducted. Stabilizing hip posteriorly, adduct hip to maximum stretch position.
Hamstrings	Toe-touching in standing or seated position with the knees straight.	Patient supine, hip flexed, knee extended, elevate leg to maximum stretch position.
Heel cords	Stand arm's length from a wall. Supporting body with hands on wall and keeping knees extended and *heels on the floor* attempt to lean chest to wall, thus dorsiflexing ankles.	Patient supine, knees extended. Cup heel in palm, maintaining foot in neutral position and supporting sole to avoid bending foot at tarsal joints. Dorsiflex ankle to position of maximal stretch.

sary for maintenance of the upright posture and proper seating when wheelchair confinement becomes necessary.

9. The patient with muscle disease should be kept orthograde for as long as possible. Standing and walking are the best functional physical therapy for accomplishing this.

   a) Two to three hours a day of such activity is encouraged.

   b) If the patient is rested after a full night's sleep, he is not being overexercised.

   c) Stretch positioning (proning) to stretch hip flexors and daily active assisted exercise can significantly lengthen the period of functional ability.

   d) Night splints are sometimes also effective in preserving joint posture.

    (1) These appliances should be used *before* deformities have occurred and in addition to, not instead of, manual contracture stretching.

    (2) Where lower extremity night splints are used, knee-ankle-foot orthoses (KAFO) are advised as AFO night splints may initiate or increase knee flexion contracture because of the tendency of patients to flex their knees in order to relieve discomfort from heel cord tightness.

  e) Patients with DMD suffer severe disuse atrophy when immobile.

    (1) Bed or chair confinement should be for no more than a day at most.

    (2) Alternate haunch standing is encouraged to avoid heel cord contracture.

    (3) Although weakening is symmetric in many of the muscular dystrophies, joint contractures are not so.

       (a) Unequal contracture occurs secondary to habitually maintained postures and also to decreased activity in nondominant extremities.

       (b) Two-joint muscles contract the earliest and the most.

BIBLIOGRAPHY

Archibald KC, Vignos PJ, Jr: A study of contractures in muscular dystrophy. *Arch Phys Med Rehabil* 1959; 40:150–157.

Cherry DB: Transfer techniques for children with muscular dystrophy. *Phys Ther* 1973; 53:970–971.

Daniels L, Williams M, Worthingham C: *Muscle Testing: Techniques of Manual Examination.* Philadelphia, WB Saunders Co, 1974.

Demos J: Early diagnosis and treatment of rapidly developing Duchenne De-Boulogne type myopathy (Type DDB 1). *Am J Phys Med* 1971; 50:271–284.

Dubowitz V: Prevention of deformities. *Isr J Med Sci* 1977; 13:183–188.

Dubowitz V, Heckmatt J: Management of muscular dystrophy; Pharmacological and physical aspects. *Br Med Bull* 1980; 36:139–144.

Florence JM, Brooke MH, Carroll JE: Evaluation of the child with muscular weakness. *Orthop Clin North Am* 1978; 9:409–430.

Fowler WM, Jr, Taylor M: Rehabilitation management of muscular dystrophy and related disorders: 1. The role of exercise. *Arch Phys Med Rehabil* 1982; 63:319–321.

Gordon EE, Texidor TA: Problems in muscle biopsy: An experimental study. *Arch Phys Med Rehabil* 1964; 45:396–402.

Hall DC, Vignos PJ, Jr: Clothing adaptations for the child with progressive muscular dystrophy. *Am J Occup Ther* 1964; 18:108–112.

Harris SE, Cherry DB: Childhood progressive muscular dystrophy and the role of physical therapy. *Phys Ther* 1974; 54:4–12.

Hoberman M: Physical medicine and rehabilitation: Its value and limitations in progressive muscular dystrophy. *Am J Phys Med Rehabil* 1955; 34: 109–115.

Hsu JD, Perry RE, Gonzales V, et al: Functional abilities of the muscle disease patient. Presented at the annual meeting of the American Academy of Orthopedic Surgeons, San Francisco, 1975.

Johnson EW, Braddom R: Overwork weakness in facioscapulohumeral muscular dystrophy. *Arch Phys Med Rehabil* 1971; 52:333–336.

Johnson EW, Kennedy JH: Comprehensive management of Duchenne muscular dystrophy. *Arch Phys Med Rehabil* 1971; 52:110–114.

Kenrick MM: Certain aspects of managing patients with muscular dystrophy. *South Med J* 1965; 58:996–1000.

Kottke FJ: The effects of limitation of activity upon the human body. JAMA 1966; 196:117–120.

Miller J: Assessment in the treatment of muscle disease (A preliminary report). *Tex Rep Biol Med* 1964; 22:871–879.

Morris AG, Vignos PJ, Jr: A self-care program for the child with progressive muscular dystrophy. *Am J Occup Ther* 1960; 14(6):301–305.

Paul WD: Medical management of contractures in muscular dystrophy. Symposium on contracture of muscle. Third Medical Conference, Muscular Dystrophy Association of America, Inc., New York, 1954.

Scott DM, Goddard C, Dubowitz V: Quantitation of muscle function in children: A prospective study in Duchenne muscular dystrophy. *Muscle Nerve* 1982; 5:291–301.

Siegel IM: Orthopedic correction of musculoskeletal deformity in muscular dystrophy, in Griggs RC, Moxley RT, III (eds): *Advances in Neurology,* vol 17. *Treatment of Neuromuscular Diseases.* New York, Raven Press, 1973, pp 343–364.

Sockolov R, Irwin B, Dressendorfer RH, et al: Exercise performance in 6- to 11-year-old boys with Duchenne muscular dystrophy. *Arch Phys Med Rehabil* 1977; 58:195–201.

Swinyard CA, Deaver GG, Greenspan L: Progressive muscular dystrophy— diagnosis and problems of rehabilitation. Science Department, Muscular Dystrophy Association of America, Inc, 1958.

Vignos PJ, Jr: Rehabilitation in progressive muscular dystrophy, in Licht S (ed): *Rehabilitation and Medicine.* New Haven, Elizabeth Licht, Publisher, 1968, pp 584–642.

Vignos PJ, Jr, Watkins MP: The effect of exercise in muscular dystrophy. *JAMA* 1966; 197:843–848.

Wratney JJ: Physical therapy for children. *Phys Ther Rev* 1958; 38:26–32.

Ziter FA, Allsop KG, Tyler FH: Assessment of muscle strength in Duchenne muscular dystrophy. *Neurology (Minneapolis)* 1977; 27:981–984.

15

Pathomechanics

"The muscles always begin and end on the bones that touch one another, and they never begin and end on the same bone. For they would not be able to move anything unless this was itself in a state of rarity or density."

Leonardo DaVinci (1452–1519)

I. Pathomechanics.
   A. All skeletal muscle is affected in Duchenne muscular dystrophy.
   B. Weakness is first noted and most severe in those antigravity muscles serving a postural role. The work density of a muscle determines its rate and degree of degeneration. Those muscles requiring the longest periods of sustained activity degenerate first. Musculature developing first phylogenetically, even if its original function is lost, is the earliest to degenerate in disease.
      1. This leads to alteration of the dynamics of postural maintenance. Included are:
         a) The muscles of the limb girdles.
         b) The knee extensors, although ultimately only two things are needed for knee extension:
            (1) Ankle equinus from whatever cause.

191

(2) Strong hip extensors.
   c) The dorsiflexors of the ankle.
2. Muscles of the lower extremity modulate more than motivate gait.
   a) The pelvis must be maintained posterior to the hip and body weight anterior to the knee at midstance.
3. "Hanging onto" ligaments requires little more energy than a properly aligned position (Fig 15–1). It may be effective (Fig 15–2), but it is hardly efficient because it is a posture that can cause pain due to stress. It is not a position from which one is able to move with dispatch. It leaves a narrow margin of safety, since joints are forced and held at their limit in one direction.
4. As weakness progresses, gravity (the unseen muscle), always in force, causes contracture, fatigue, and eventually inhibits the upright posture.

II. Postural Dynamics.*
   A. Wasting in DMD bears a direct relationship to muscular function. The skeletal segments of the body are moving levers, powered by muscles monitored through a feedback (gamma) system. Vertical bodily displacements are against gravity and as a rule require more energy and superimpose more stress than horizontal movements.
   B. With absence of the stretch reflex, passive stretch can occur, leaving an inadequately responsive muscle vulnerable to ordinary strain.

III. Work hypertrophy is seen in the antigravity muscles maintaining postural alignment. Such postural overwork (hypertrophy) weakens the dystrophic muscle. Such muscles are:
   A. Buttocks, thighs, and calves in the lower extremities and shoulder stabilizers in the upper.
   B. Serratus anterior is a major postural fixator of the shoulder and affected early. Regional differences relate to:
   1. Postural, supportive, and traumatic factors.
      a) A dynamic postural role of muscle is served by reflex contractile responses. During locomotion, these reflexes control the position of various body segments with respect to each other and bring about proper orientation of the body in space.

*"Motion is modified posture . . . posture accompanies movement like a shadow . . . every movement begins and ends in posture. . ." C. S. Sherrington (1857–1952).

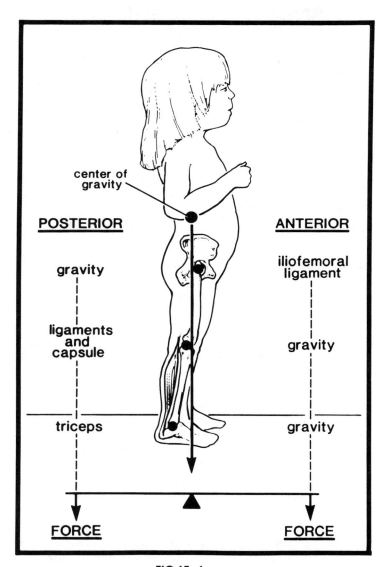

FIG 15–1.
Balance vector.

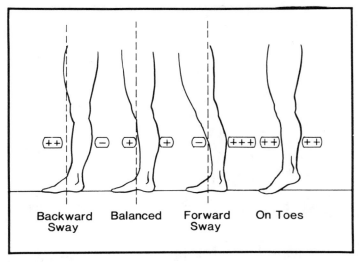

FIG 15–2.
Below knee muscle activity. (Modified from Basmajian JV: *Muscles Alive: Their Functions Revealed by Electromyography,* ed 2. Baltimore, Williams & Wilkins Co, 1967. Used by permission.)

          b) As the disease advances, reflex function is lost (the muscle spindle becomes "detuned"), functional muscle mass is reduced, and the muscle deteriorates.

          c) Finally, the muscle subserves only a passive supportive role.

            (1) Thus, dynamic (kinetic) stability degenerates to passive (static) stability, which finally weakens to instability.

            (2) With decline in elasticity and reflex contractility, muscle is now vulnerable to deforming forces imposed by postural or supportive traumatic stress (Fig 15–3). Such stress can be active, such as that put upon the gastrocnemius during overwork, or passive, like the stretching of pectoralis major in maintaining torso balance.

    2. Although physiologically at rest, muscle is physically in a state of tonic stretch. Muscle spindles protect against overstretch. Loss of its deep tendon reflex marks the regression of a muscle from a kinetic to a static state.

  C. Psoas (postural) is more severely involved than iliacus (nonpostural).

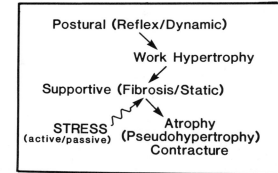

FIG 15–3.
Differential muscle atrophy.

    D. Abdominal portion of pectoralis major is more involved than its clavicular segment.

    E. Clavicular head of sternocleidomastoid suffers more than the sternal component.

IV. Normal locomotion requires modulation of the center of gravity just anterior to the lumbosacral junction. Additionally, the initiation of gait is superintended by a finely tuned neuromuscular mechanism, permitting the center of gravity to move posteriorly and toward the limb that is to swing and then onto the one that is to be the stance limb. The body then proceeds to take the first step.

    A. Walking has been compared to a controlled fall. Normal locomotion translates the center of gravity through space along a path requiring minimal energy expenditure (Fig 15–4). The center of gravity is elevated in the stance phase of gait, thus building potential energy. This is converted to kinetic energy during swing phase.

    B. Some vertical center of gravity displacement is necessary to achieve this potential-kinetic energy trade-off (approximately 5 cm). Unproductive movement is balanced off by certain coordinated joint motions (Fig 15–5), including:

        1. Pelvic rotation of 5 degrees.

        2. Pelvic tilt of 5 cm on swing side.

        3. Knee flexion on stance leg.

        4. Coupling of knee extension with ankle dorsiflexion and knee flexion with ankle plantar flexion (Fig 15–6), maintaining equal leg length throughout gait.

        5. Physiologic knee valgus (Fig 15–7) placing foot under center of gravity without excessive lateral torso shift during stance.

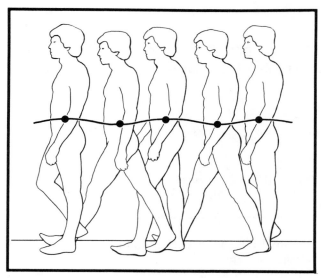

FIG 15–4.
Center of gravity displacement during normal gait.

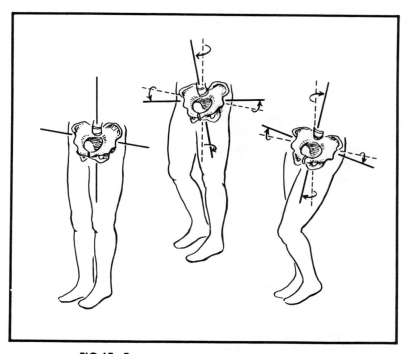

FIG 15–5.
Rotation of the pelvis, pelvic tilt, and knee flexion.

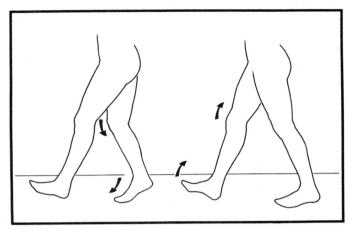

FIG 15—6.
Knee and ankle coupling motions.

C. Such postural adaptations enable the body to remain upright by maintaining the line of the center of gravity within its base of support. They also cause the center of body mass to move at uniform velocity along a low amplitude sine-wave path with minimal energy consumption.

D. Newton's third law (each action is opposed by an opposite and equal reaction) is served as the torque of ground contact (Fig 15–8) during gait passes upward through the center of gravity, avoiding undue angular acceleration of the body when in motion.

E. The Duchenne dystrophic cannot control momentary imbalances imposed by competing demands for both knee and hip stability. Such adjustments are increasingly difficult as weakness and contracture progress. The trunk represents 70% of the body's weight. Steadying it over the pelvis becomes a progressively arduous task. Postural status regresses from stability to merely balance and finally to imbalance and instability.

1. Muscular dystrophy patients lose the ability to control the momentary imbalances that occur in normal locomotion. This is due to progressive:

    a) Weakness.

    b) Contracture.

    c) Loss of muscle spindle proprioceptive function resulting in an attempt to preserve as minimal a level of energy

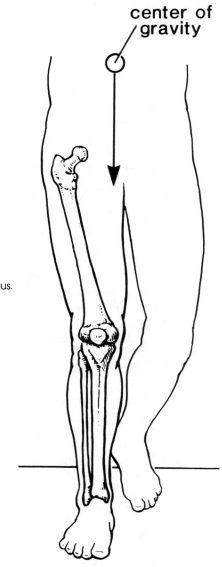

FIG 15–7.
Normal knee valgus.

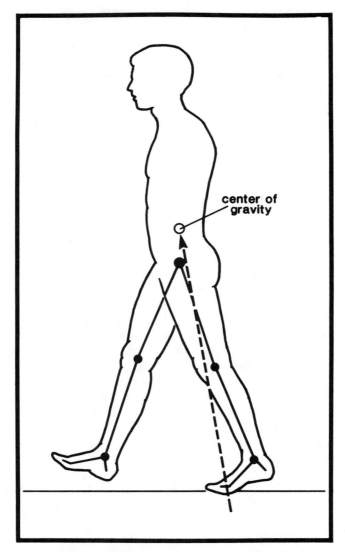

FIG 15—8.
Ground reaction force vector.

expenditure as possible through exaggerations of motion at unaffected, or less affected, body levels. Also, in order to maintain balance, multiple groups of postural muscles may act out of their expected phase.

V. Clinical correlation—biokinetics.

    A. In DMD, hip flexors, tensor fasciae latae, and triceps surae develop ambulation limiting contractures.

        1. Contractures are seldom symmetrical and seem to be greater on the nondominant side.

        2. Quadriceps insufficiency is the key factor in gait deterioration.

        3. The earliest postural change in the lower extremities is an increase in lumbar lordosis secondary to gluteus maximus weakness (Fig 15–9) (the upper half of this muscle has an abduction function; the lower half is pure extensor). Hip extension at this time is largely performed by the hamstring muscles.

        4. Some changes in joint lever systems occur. For instance, the hip is a first class lever with force exerted by the abductors over the fulcrum of the articulated femoral head to balance body weight (Fig 15–10). As hip abductors weaken, hip hikers (quadratus lumborum) are called upon to elevate the hip during swing, thus creating a third class lever, where power is sacrificed for a wider arc of movement.

    B. With progression of quadriceps weakness, hip adductors are called upon to assist knee extension. As contracture increases, the base of support decreases, pelvic-femoral alignment is unstabilized, and the patient can no longer utilize normal postural mechanisms for efficient balance. He must walk with a wide gait, characterized by:

        1. Equinus posturing caused by forward shift of the center of gravity (Fig 15–11), which now falls anterior to a point 60% of foot length (measured from heel to toe) as contrasted with 40% in the normal.

        2. Heel varus.

        3. Knee flexion, in an effort to lower the center of gravity for better balance (the lower a body's CG, the longer the arc required to displace it) (Fig 15–12), aggravated by both tensor fascia and hip flexion contractures.

        4. Hip flexion.

        5. Hip abduction (Fig 15–13).

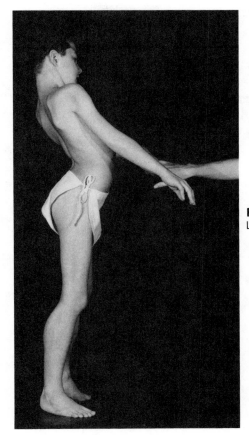

FIG 15–9.
Lumbar lordosis.

C. Exaggerated lumbar lordosis is a functional deformity noted early as the patient attempts to compensate for pelvic force imbalance secondary to weakened hip extension, accompanied by hip flexion contracture. Abdominal muscle weakness allows the pelvis to drop anteriorly, augmenting this deformity.
D. In lordosis, the center of gravity is shifted posteriorly. The child adjusts by rising on the balls of his feet and ultimately onto his toes. Some equinus is necessary to compensate for the displacement of the CG as well as weakness of the quadriceps.
E. Abdominal and low back extensor weakness contribute to this awkward and effortful posture as loss of scapular stabilizer

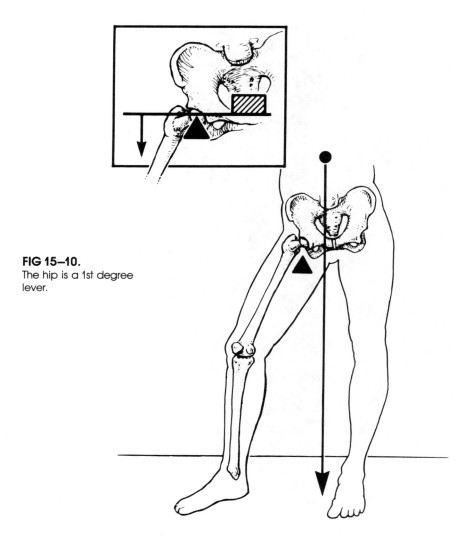

FIG 15–10.
The hip is a 1st degree lever.

strength draws the shoulders forward, requiring exaggerated lumbar lordosis to achieve torso balance. The torque tending to flex the knee is aggravated by increasing lumbar lordosis as the tendency of the hip flexors to flex the hip also flexes (unlocks) the knee.

F. Hips are further abducted in an effort to widen the base of support so that the line of gravity will fall within its confines.

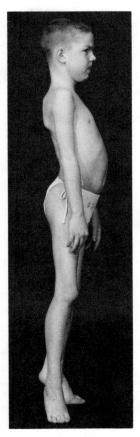

FIG 15–11.
Equinus.

G. Several biarticular muscles of the lower extremity, functioning within a closed kinetic chain, may reverse their usual roles in response to the antigravity needs of this postural crisis.
   1. With fixed equinus (Fig 15–14), the soleus (sometimes gastrocnemius) functions as an extensor of the knee. With the ankle fixed in equinus and hip extension prevented by a superincumbent body load, the hamstrings will contract in a vain attempt to extend the knee and keep the body upright.
H. The long arch is obliterated secondary to early minimal heel cord contracture. It is reconstructed with the initiation of inevitable equinovarus deformity.

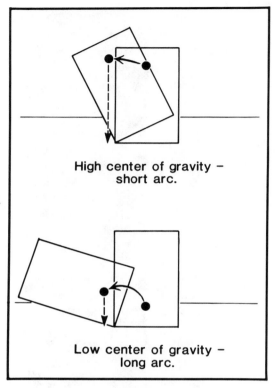

High center of gravity –
short arc.

FIG 15–12.
Solid body displacement.

Low center of gravity –
long arc.

I. As the ankle is held in plantar flexion, the narrow portion of the talus (Fig 15–15) is brought into the mortise, rendering this joint vulnerable to those forces shaping a rotatory deformity (e.g., the foot may invert at the initiation of stance).

J. The center of hip rotation shifts medially during standing. Psoas major functions as an external hip rotator in swing phase and an internal rotator during stance. Tensor fasciae latae internally rotates the hip. Reasonable agonist-antagonist rotation balance is maintained at the hip joint, and severe rotational deformities are not usually seen in ambulatory Duchenne muscular dystrophy. As the disease progresses, the lower extremities are progressively externally rotated to widen the base of support. A small subset of children, instead of rotating the hip out, exhibit hip joint valgus and anteversion with internal rotation of the legs. This effectively medially rotates the knee joints out of the plane of flexion buckling, and

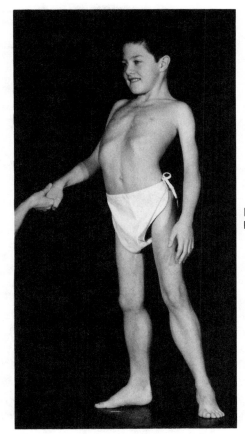

FIG 15–13.
Hip abduction.

the hip extensor force of the adductor magnus and hamstrings can assist knee extension. The adductor-hamstring extensor response is apparently facilitated through reflexes of the gait pattern rather than being called on as prime movers. Additionally, as an active (though weak) internal hip rotator, tensor fascia also aids this process.

K. Ultimately the head is used as an adjustment force. As the trunk is maintained in extension, the neck is held flexed. This delicate balance permits proper positioning of the weight line behind the hips and in front of the knees.

L. Hip extension ability finally determines whether or not a patient will walk. The knee and the foot can be braced, but (except for the reciprocal dynamic extension orthosis useful in

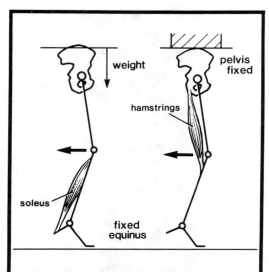

FIG 15–14.
Closed kinetic chain.

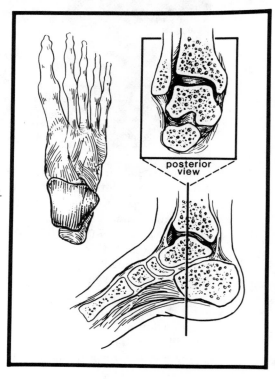

FIG 15–15.
Equinus instability.

highly selected cases with essentially flail hips with some residual hip hiker strength) there is no effective ambulatory
brace for the weak hip.

ENERGETICS

I. As long as the patient can maintain the line of gravity behind
his hips, in front of the knees, and within his base of support,
he can stand upright (Fig 15–16). Compensatory mechanisms
(lordosis, equinus, hip abduction) provide simultaneous hip and
knee stability for awhile (Fig 15–17). Leaning back stabilizes the
hips when gluteus maximus is weak; leaning forward locks the
knees when quadriceps is weak. A precarious balance must be
maintained between these two competing postural demands. As
the safe movement range narrows, increasing effort is required
for ambulation. Falling and the fear of losing balance also inhibit
walking.
II. Gait requires body unbalancing through the coordinated activity
of tibialis anticus, quadriceps, hip abductors and peroneal muscles, a process the Duchenne dystrophic patient finds difficult to
perform.
III. To execute the swing phase of gait, the hip must extend and the
extensor muscles unload.
   A. Progressive hip flexion contracture in DMD interferes with

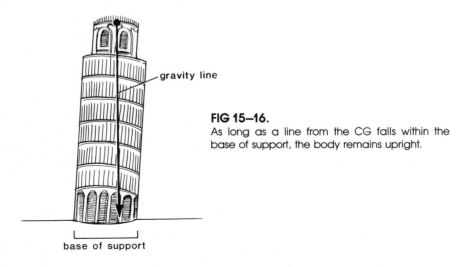

gravity line

FIG 15–16.
As long as a line from the CG falls within the
base of support, the body remains upright.

base of support

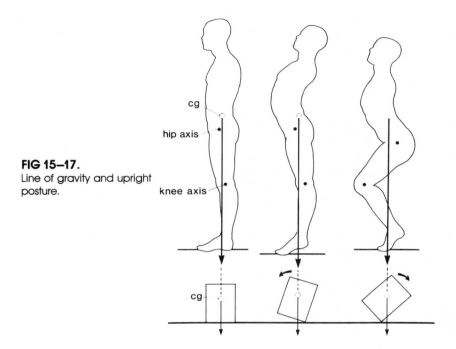

FIG 15–17.
Line of gravity and upright posture.

both these requisites. Weakened erector spinae and hip abductors cannot adequately elevate the swing hip.

IV. Inability to properly modulate the center of gravity during gait, utilizing normal compensatory mechanisms to minimize energy expenditure in forward motion, and inability to balance the ground reaction through proper control of angular acceleration lead to excessive rolling of the body for balance in DMD at a severe expenditure of metabolic energy during ambulation.

V. The most severe contractures occur in postural muscles spanning two joints.

VI. Muscular weakness, tendon contracture, and mechanical malposture contribute to ultimate deformity

VII. An outline of the biomechanical sequence leading to the typical dystrophic posture (Fig 15–18) is as follows:*

  A. Hip extensor and shoulder stabilizer weakness.

  B. Hip flexor contracture, thrusting the trunk forward.

  C. Compensatory lumbar lordosis.

*Progression of weakness, contracture, and deformity in various muscle groups is not entirely sequential. These events overlap, and some occur concurrently.

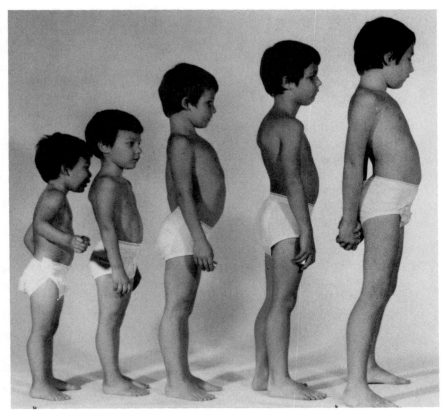

FIG 15–18.
DMD in five siblings. Note progressive lordosis, hip abduction, equinus, and shoulder and head thrust necessary for balance.

  D. Forward shift of center of mass forcing patient to rise on toes, thus shortening ankle-to-toes lever arm and shifting center of gravity forward.
  E. Hip abduction to increase equilibrium by widening body's base of support.
  F. Secondary tensor fasciae latae contractures.
  G. External tibial torsion; thus, ankle and knee axes are no longer in the same plane.
  H. Ankle varus (an effort to bring ankle and foot into better postural alignment).
  I. Mild knee flexion to lower center of mass and gain balance.

    J. Progressive quadriceps weakness requiring equinus to lock knees for stability.

    K. With foot fixed in equinus and knee flexed, gastrocnemius and soleus can now act to extend knee.

    L. True overwork exercise hypertrophy of calves.

    M. Widening of base of support with concomitant increase of those forces causing equinocavovarus.

        1. Unopposed heel-cord contracture acting upon eccentric medial insertion of Achilles tendon.

        2. Tarsal slide in an anterior and medial direction.

        3. Increase of toe-flexion action for grasp stability.

        4. Secondary intrinsic foot muscle contracture.

        5. Unopposed action of tibialis posticus against weak peroneals and tibialis anticus.

        6. Strong toe flexors working against weakened toe extensors.

    N. Triceps surae overwork with "pseudohypertrophy."

VIII. The result of these events is a stance and gait typified by the following descriptors (Fig 15–19):†

    A. Hip flexion and abduction.

    B. Increasing lumbar lordosis.

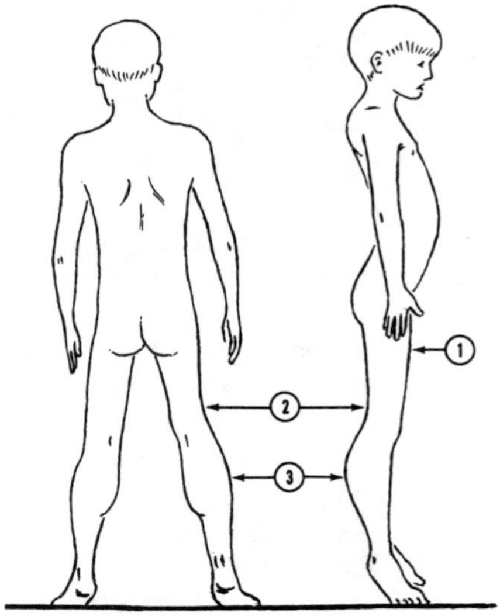

FIG 15–19.
Stance and gait typified by lumbar lordosis due to *(1)* hip flexion, *(2)* hip abduction with ankle equinus secondary to contracture of *(3)* gastrocsoleus.

†One should distinguish between primary deformity (e.g., hip extensor weakness), secondary deformity (e.g., hip flexor contracture), and compensatory deformity (e.g., hip abduction, lumbar lordosis, and ankle equinus) in planning therapy.

TABLE 15–1.
Causes of Ambulatory Loss in DMD

Predisposing: progressive weakness, wasting, contracture
Precipitating: uncompensated malposture with growth (ht/wt)
Perpetuating: inability to properly modulate CG, leading to instability

    C. Foot equinocavovarus.
 IX. Mediolateral subtalar instability secondary to muscle imbalance (strong posterior tibial, weak peroneals, etc.) allows the foot to invert during the swing phase of gait.
    A. Initiation of stance in this insecure position may cause falling.
  X. Generalized weakness makes it increasingly difficult to attain alignment stability when the trunk is balanced over unstable lower extremities (Table 15–1).

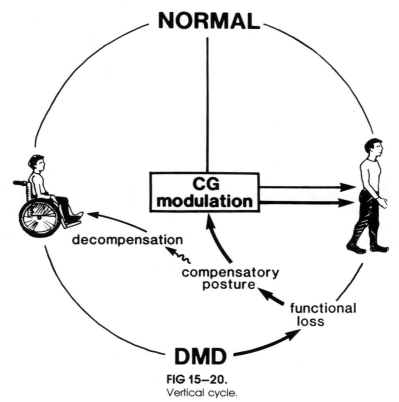

FIG 15–20.
Vertical cycle.

XI. Proprioceptive abilities are also affected.
XII. Sufficient strength to execute those postural adjustments necessary to compensate for weakening and contracture is lacking.
Postural adaptations are most often achieved by altering the in-
tensity of muscular contraction rather than by changes in phasic
activity.
   A. Small nonmuscular changes assume significance. A slight
      weight gain or a period of several days of bedrest can de-
      crease strength enough to impair ambulation. In its later
      stages, DMD is a brittle disease, and the transition from
      moderately to severely impaired ambulation may be abrupt.
   B. Because of individual differences in weakness, contracture,
      weight, and motivation, age alone is a poor index of disease
      progression.
   C. The more disabled the patient, the more determinants of
      gait are lost, the more energy is required for ambulation,
      and the less efficient is the gait (Fig 15–20).

BIBLIOGRAPHY

Bonsett CA: Studies of pseudohypertrophic muscular dystrophy. Springfield,
   Illinois, Charles C Thomas, Publisher, 1969.
Bonsett CA: Prophylactic bracing in pseudohypertrophic muscular dystrophy.
   Indiana Med 1975; 68:181–184.
Bowker JH, Halpin PJ: Factors determining success in reambulation of the
   child with progressive muscular dystrophy. *Orthop Clin North Am* 1978;
   9:431–436.
Cochran G, Van B: *A Primer of Orthopaedic Biomechanics.* New York, Churchill
   Livingstone, Inc, 1982.
Curtis BH: Orthopaedic management of muscular dystrophy and related dis-
   orders, in *AAOS: Instructional Course Lectures,* no 19. St Louis, CV Mosby
   Co, 1970, pp 78–89.
Edelstein G: Correlation of handedness and degree of joint contracture in bi-
   lateral muscle and joint disease. *Am J Phys Med* 1959; 38:45–47.
Fisher SV, Gullickson G, Jr: Energy cost of ambulation in health and disabil-
   ity: A literature review. *Arch Phys Med Rehabil* 1978; 59:124–133.
Galasko CSB: Incidence of orthopedic problems in children with muscle dis-
   ease. *Isr J Med Sci* 1977; 13:165–176.
Gucker T: Muscular dystrophy. *Phys Ther* 1964; 44:243–246.
Huddleston OL: Postural reflexes. *Arch Phys Ther* 1940; 21:282–289.
Johnson EW: Pathokinesiology of Duchenne muscular dystrophy: Implications
   of management. *Arch Phys Med Rehabil* 1977; 58:4–7.

Johnson EW, Kennedy JH: Comprehensive management of Duchenne muscular dystrophy. *Arch Phys Med Rehabil* 1971; 52:110–114.

Mann EA, Hagy JL, White V, et al: The initiation of gait. *J Bone Joint Surg* 1979; 61A(2):232–234.

Melkonian DVM, Cristofaro RL, Perry J, et al: Dynamic gait electromyography study in Duchenne muscular dystrophy (DMD) patients. *Foot Ankle* 1980; 1:78–83.

Merton PA: How we control the contraction of our muscles. *Sci Am* 1972; 226:30–37.

Pearson K: The control of walking. *Sci Am* 1976; 235(6):72–74.

Pohtilla JF: Kinesiology of hip extension at selected angles of pelvifemoral extension. *Arch Phys Med Rehabil* 1969; 50:241–250.

Radin E, Simon S, Rose R, et al: *Practical Biomechanics for the Orthopedic Surgeon.* New York, John Wiley & Sons, 1979.

Rosenthal AM: Normal and abnormal gait patterns. *IMJ* 1969; 136:50–54.

Seeger BR, Caudrey DJ, Little JD: Progression of equinus deformity in Duchenne muscular dystrophy. *Arch Phys Med Rehabil* 1985; 66:286–288.

Siegel IM: Pathomechanics of stance in Duchenne muscular dystrophy. *Arch Phys Med Rehabil* 1972; 53:403–406.

Siegel IM: Postural substitution in Duchenne's muscular dystrophy. *JAMA* 1982; 247:584.

Sutherland DH, Olshen R, Cooper L, et al: The pathomechanics of gait in Duchenne muscular dystrophy. *Dev Med Child Neurol* 1981; 23:3–22.

Waters RL, Hislop HJ, Perry J, et al: Energetics: Application to the study and management of locomotor disabilities: Energy cost of normal and pathologic gait. *Orthop Clin North Am* 1978; 9:351–356.

16

Treatment: General Remarks

"Use strengthens, disuse debilitates."
Hippocrates (460?–377? B.C.), *The Surgery XX*
(Translated by E.T. Withington)

I. Optimal treatment for the patient with a muscle disease should be:
   A. Prospective.
   B. Aggressive.
   C. Conducted in an atmosphere of intelligent concern.
II. Total management is best administered by a team that includes a:
   A. Pediatrician.
   B. Neurologist.
   C. Geneticist.
   D. Physiatrist.
   E. Orthopedic consultant.
   F. In addition, the following personnel can assist the patient and family:
      1. Physical therapist.
      2. Occupational therapist.
      3. Medical social worker or psychologist.
      4. Dietician.
      5. Respiratory therapist.

6. Speech therapist.
7. Subspecialty consultant (i.e., gastrointestinal, cardiopulmonary, etc).

III. Surgical treatment. The aim of surgery is to release ambulation limiting contractures sufficiently to maintain adequate standing and walking equilibrium. In order to do this, appropriate orthoses offering satisfactory support without undue weight are prescribed after surgery.

A. Surgical intervention is indicated at appropriate times in the natural progression of the disease.

1. Most patients with DMD stop walking between 9–12 years of age. The ectomorphic child usually walks (and reambulates after surgery) for a longer time than his endomorphic counterpart.

2. The ability to easily rise from a seated position, ascend stairs, and walk are usually lost in that sequence at yearly intervals.

3. When the sum of the knee extension lag and hip extension lag reaches 90 degrees in the face of ankle equinus of 15 degrees or more (Fig 16–1), the child can no longer maintain the upright posture, and ambulation soon ends. In this regard, the patient can usually tolerate knee extension lag better than extension lag of the hip because with fixed ankle equinus the knee (a hinge joint) can be locked into stable extension, whereas the hip (a ball and socket joint) cannot.

B. Surgical management must permit early postoperative mobilization. Even brief restraint can lead to rapid loss of strength. Several factors may prove useful in prognosticating ambulating success with surgery and bracing. These include (in combination):

1. Percentage of residual muscle strength at the time of operation.

2. Vital capacity (an excellent reflection of overall residual strength).

3. Patient motivation.

4. Creatinine coefficient and its decrease in the several years just before surgery. This last biochemical index is linked to increased creatine, decreased creatinine excretion (urinary excretion of these compounds is related in reciprocal fashion, and creatine/creatinine ratio and creatine tolerance testing [though nonspecific] can be used in the diagnosis of

HIP EXTENSION LAG

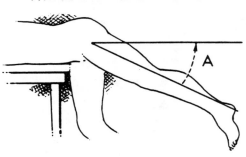

FIG 16–1.

KNEE EXTENSION LAG

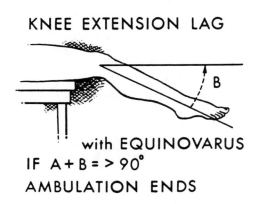

with EQUINOVARUS
IF A + B = > 90°
AMBULATION ENDS

neuromuscular disease). Creatinine excretion directly reflects functional muscle mass. The creatinine coefficient relates 24-hour urinary excretion to body weight (mg/kg) and decreases as myopathy progresses and muscle mass decreases.

C. Once a patient is wheelchair-confined, it is difficult, if not impossible, to regain the ability to stand and walk.

D. Anesthesia. Patients with muscle disease are poor anesthetic risks.
1. They have inadequate pulmonary reserve and require an impeccable airway during anesthesia.
2. They may run the risk of malignant hyperthermia.
3. Depolarizing agents may cause a sharp rise in serum potassium, placing the patient at increased jeopardy for cardiac arrest.

4. Serum creatine phosphokinase is elevated in the intraoperative period.
5. Respiratory failure increases with exposure to depressive drugs.
6. Anesthesia must be closely monitored, paying particular attention to:
    a) Adequate ventilation.
    b) Preventing gastric dilatation.
    c) Prohibiting potassium overload.
    d) Close cardiac monitoring.

BIBLIOGRAPHY

Cobham IG, Davis HS: Anesthesia for muscle dystrophy patients. *Anesth Analg* 1964; 43:22–29.

Cohen PJ: Halogenated anesthetic and patients with elevated CPK level. *JAMA* (Questions and Answers) 1972; 220:1253.

Fowler WM, Jr: Medical rehabilitation of persons with muscular dystrophy and other neuromuscular disorders. Rehabilitation Research Review, NARIC, NCRI, Data Institute, The Catholic University of America, Washington, DC, 1985.

Isaacs H, Barlow B: Malignant hyperpyrexia: Further muscle studies in asymptomatic carriers identified by creatine phosphokinase screening. *J Neurol Neurosurg Psychiatry* 1973; 36:228–243.

Siegel IM: *The Clinical Management of Muscle Disease.* London, William Heinemann Medical Books Ltd, 1977.

Vignos PJ, Jr: Physical models of rehabilitation in neuromuscular disease. *Muscle Nerve* 1983; 6:323–338.

17

Surgery and Bracing: Lower Extremity

"The feasibility of an operation is not the best indication for its performance."

Henry, Lord Cohen of Birkenhend (1900–)

I. Maintenance of the upright posture and ambulation (either community or household) can be extended from two to four years beyond the time it would ordinarily cease by lower extremity contracture release and appropriate bracing. This treatment may add both years to the patient's life as well as life to his remaining years.
   A. Percutaneous release of heel cords, iliotibial band, (bipolar tensor fascia, if distal release inadequate) and superficial hip flexors (when degree of hip flexion contracture prevents torsopelvic balance in spite of tensor fascia release), followed by appropriate plaster casts and subsequent bracing will allow the patient to be up the day of surgery and walking the next (Fig 17–1).
      1. These procedures are indicated when the sum of hip and knee extension lag reaches 90 degrees. Cessation of ambu-

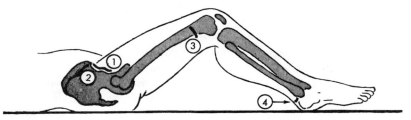

FIG 17–1.
Sites of percutaneous contracture release: *(1)* hip flexors, *(2)* and *(3)* bipolar tensor fascia, and *(4)* Achilles tendon.

lation is usually heralded by decreased upright stability and increased falling. Hip abductor strength and absence of severe fixed lower extremity deformity seem to predict a successful surgical result.

2. Subcutaneous tenotomy of hip flexors (including sartorius and straight head of rectus femoris) is accomplished by introducing a tenotome at the anterior-superior iliac spine and sweeping it distally and posteriorly. The knife is kept close to bone and the procedure performed while the contralateral hip is fully flexed. Flexion contracture can usually be decreased by at least 50%. Remaining contracture exists in the deeper hip flexors (iliopsoas) as well as the anterior hip capsule.

3. Through the same stab wound, the tenotome severs the origin of tensor fasciae latae at the lateral aspect of the anterior portion of the iliac crest.

4. Bipolar tensor fasciae tenotomy is completed by subcutaneous release of the iliotibial band just proximal to the lateral aspect of the knee joint. Section of the lateral intermuscular septum (necessary because the iliotibial band inserts there) is assured when this incision is carried to bone. Separation of approximately 2.5 cm in the palpable ends of the transected iliotibial band, accompanied by correction of tensor fasciae latae contracture, is accomplished.

5. Percutaneous tenotomy of the heel cord is performed in its distal third.*

*Heel cord lengthening as an isolated procedure will not succeed if the quadriceps is weak, unless accompanied by long leg bracing. It is sometimes utilized (along with isolated iliotibial band release) in the young child (7 years of age) if the quadriceps is graded fair or better. Under these circumstances, a below-knee orthosis (AFO) modified for floor reaction is prescribed postoperatively.

a) Release of the Achilles tendon is carried out without a tourniquet because a tourniquet may prevent hematoma localization by permitting skin to fall into the space created by separation of the cut ends of the tendon. With the patient supine, a fine tenotome is introduced through a stab wound just medial to the dorsal surface of the insertion of the tendo Achillis. The knife enters in a longitudinal direction through the medial wound. The blade is directed toward the dorsal surface of the tendon, stretching the skin as it proceeds. This allows the stab wound to lie away from the transected tendon when the skin retracts after the procedure. The blade is then rotated 90 degrees so that its cutting edge faces the tendon's posterior surface. It is important to keep the blade on the tendon to avoid cutting either the skin or its underlying supporting layer of tissue; otherwise, a skin slough may develop. The ankle is dorsiflexed while pressure is placed on the blade. Only pressure, not a "sawing motion," is used, allowing the tendon to "cut itself" on the blade. One-half to two-thirds of the cross-section of the tendon is transected. The tenotome is removed. On forceful dorsiflexion of the ankle, the remainder of the tendon stretches or tears, correcting the equinus deformity. A small dressing is placed on the wound (occasionally, a single 3–0 plain catgut suture is necessary).

6. Either posterior tibial transfer or release can be utilized (prophylactically) in the younger patient. This obviates the deforming force of the tibialis posticus.* The transferred muscle is often active on command but not in phase. It loses a grade in transfer. Nonetheless, even if it functions only as an active tenodesis, progressive inversion deformation can often be avoided. Transfer can be routed through the interosseous membrane to the dorsum of the foot (Fig 17–2).

7. Toe to groin light casts of plaster or plastic are applied with the ankles at neutral and the knees in 5 degrees of flexion. If there is more than 5-degree knee flexion contracture prior to surgery, it is stretched out with serial or wedging casts. Surgical correction of knee contractures has not been

*The posterior tibial muscle has a strength percentage greater than the anterior tibial or peroneus longus and exceeded only by the soleus and medial gastrocnemius.

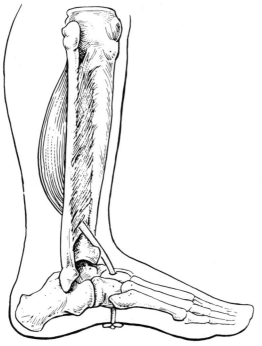

FIG 17–2.
Posterior tibial transfer.

found necessary, though release of tensor fasciae concomitantly corrects some knee flexion.

a) The plantar surfaces of the plaster are flattened on a board during application.

b) The heels of the casts are lined with sheepskin and split and spread to avoid pressure (Fig 17–3).

c) The bottoms of the casts are pounded soft and adhesive tape applied to the soles for friction. This is more stable than rubber walkers and provides firmer floor contact, reinforcing the body's kinesthetic supporting response.

d) The casts are worn for three weeks, and then knee-ankle-foot orthoses are fitted. As the patient grows, braces require lengthening, or pelvic imbalance will cause lumbar kyphosis (Fig 17–4). However, care must be taken not to bring the proximal support higher than 2 cm below the ischial tuberosity, or the orthoses will not permit the ischial support necessary for ambulation.

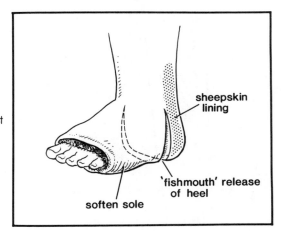

FIG 17–3.
Postoperative cast modifications.

sheepskin lining

'fishmouth' release of heel

soften sole

B. Orthoses.
    1. All orthoses are vacuum-molded plastic (Fig 17–5). Muscle activity, of course, is minimal when orthoses are used. Features of some common orthotic plastics are listed in Table 17–1.
        a) These are considerably lighter but as sturdy as their steel or aluminum counterparts.
        b) The plastic brace (Fig 17–6) incorporates a molded foot plate that obviates the need for an attached orthotic shoe. Any footwear, even tennis or running shoes (the most desirable shoe for such patients because of their lightness and soles, which grip the floor), can be comfortably worn with such a brace.
        c) Ankle mobility can be regulated by varying the width of the posterior strut connecting the calf portion to the foot plate.
        d) The appliance is form fitted from plastic and thus less bulky than a standard brace, more comfortable, and cosmetically acceptable. It can be worn under an ordinary stocking and does not require special clothing adaptations.
        e) Velcro fittings are used for closure, or a single tubular construction may be prescribed (Fig 17–7). This can utilize thinner copolymer because the tubular form (acting on the principle of a thin-walled pressure vessel) is more resistant to superimposed torsion stresses than the

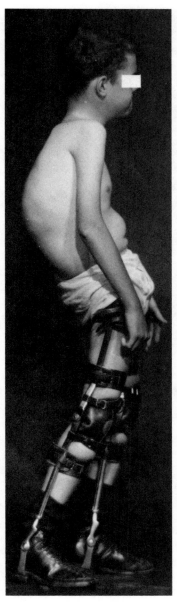

FIG 17—4.
Braces require lengthening. Note kyphosis and posturing in an attempt to keep the line of gravity behind the hips and in front of the knees.

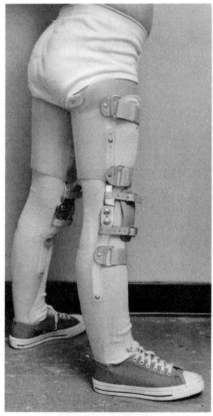

FIG 17–5.
KAFO: lateral view.

open model (Fig 17–8). Any standard knee hinge (including drop- or bail-locks) can be incorporated in the orthoses.

f) All materials used in the orthoses are nontoxic, radiolucent, unaffected by oils or ultraviolet light, and completely waterproof. The appliances can be washed and dried with ease, a characteristic contrasting with the difficulty of cleaning the leather utilized in an ordinary brace.

g) Because of their lightness, ease of application and removal, cosmetic acceptability and the other advantages enumerated above, there is strong patient compliance and parent satisfaction with these orthoses.

TABLE 17–1.
Use and Features of Some Common
Orthotic Plastics

Orthoplast (isoprene) (body jackets)
   Shapes at 160 degrees
   Lasts 9–12 months
   Cannot clean without water
Polyethylene (body jackets)
   Petrochemical
   Works at 400 degrees
   Doesn't crack
   Very flexible
   Very warm (nonporous)
   Cannot glue
Polypropylene (KAFO and AFO)
   Very light
   Very rigid
   Other properties similar to polyethylene
Plastazote (unicellular expanded polyethylene)
   Pelite aliplast (linings, inserts)
Ortholene (body jackets and extremity splints)
   Has same properties as polyethylene but alloyed with fillers
   More resistant to cracking than polyethylene
Sub-Ortholene (use as Ortholene)
   Similar to Ortholene except it has added fillers that allow
     it to be worked by a hammer
Coylene (KAFO and AFO)
   A mixture of 80% polypropylene/20% polyethylene
   Not as rigid as polypropylene
   Most resistant to cracking
Surlon
   Because it is a clear plastic, status of underlying skin can be
     easily evaluated for pressure lesions
   More flexible than polyethylene with essentially the same
     properties
Kydex
Raylon
   Rigid, used for bivalved body jackets, workable at 375
     degrees

II. Postoperative care (Table 17–2).
   A. Nasal oxygen and intermittent positive-pressure breathing.
   B. Electric circular bed, permitting the patient to stand (Fig 17–9)
      with feet resting on foot board attachment the afternoon of
      surgery.
     1. Hips stretched into extension and abduction by placing legs

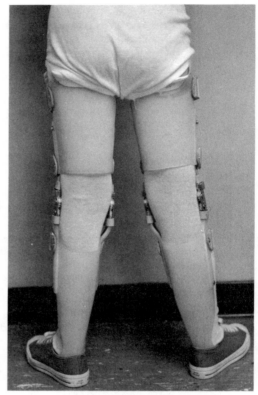

FIG 17–6.
KAFO: posterior view.

together and elevating sacrum when patient is supine and knees when he is prone (Fig 17–10,A and B).

C. Physical therapy (standing in bed and passive hip exercise) initiated the afternoon of surgery with ambulation the first postoperative day (Table 17–3). Initially, the use of a light aluminum walker may be necessary until patient adjusts to his rediscovered balance. During walking, torso shift over the supporting limb is still necessary but lumbar lordosis disappears when the patient sits and the ischial weight bearing feature of his orthoses encourage this.

D. Hospitalization for a week or less, after which a program of physical therapy including walking and hip stretching is continued at home. Braces may be worn as night splints, if tolerated.

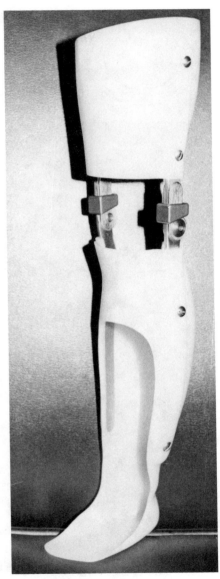

FIG 17–7.
Tubular KAFO.

FIG 17–8.
A closed cylinder is stronger because stress lines move in only one direction.

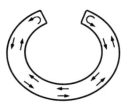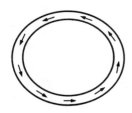

FIG 17–9.
Standing in electric circular bed.

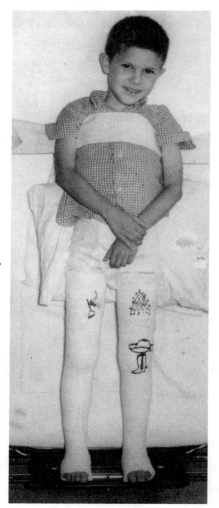

TABLE 17–2.
Postoperative Care

CircOlectric bed
Nasal oxygen
Intermittent positive pressure breathing
Standing bed position on afternoon of surgery

TABLE 17–3.
Physical Therapy Sequence

Day of surgery: passive hip stretching
First postoperative day: ambulation
Hospitalization one week: hip stretching and ambulation
Home physical therapy program continues
Braces fitted three weeks postoperatively

E. Patients continuing to walk in orthoses maintain better alignment of weight-bearing joints and suffer less sedentary osteoporosis and disuse muscular atrophy than those not ambulatory.

F. Through surgery and bracing, one can break the vicious cycle of events in muscular dystrophy (weakness-imbalance-contracture-deformity), thus delaying progression of disability.

G. Although more than half the dystrophic patient's total muscle mass is lost by the end of independent ambulation, when he is sometimes too weak to stand alone, he is often able to walk again after correction of contractures and bracing because other factors are also influential in preventing ambulation. Such causes are:
  1. Muscular atrophy secondary to decreased physical activity.
  2. Obesity.
  3. Emotional problems.
  4. Wheelchair immobilization imposed for the convenience of others.

H. Complications of percutaneous lower extremity surgery include:
  1. Heel decubitus ulcer.
    a) By split-spreading the heel portion of the cast and lining it with sheepskin, a decubitus ulcer can be avoided.
  2. Transection of superficial nerves.
    a) Occasional transection of a superficial branch of the lateral femoral cutaneous nerve results in a usually tran-

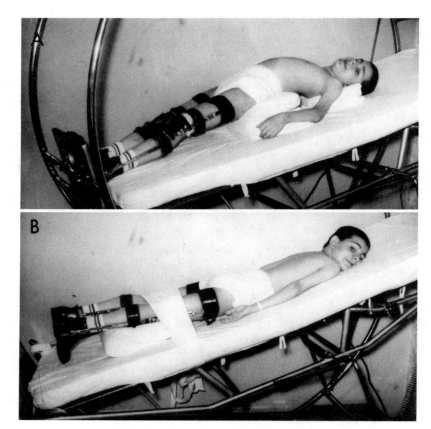

FIG 17–10.
A and **B,** passive hip stretching in bed.

sient zone of hypesthesia along the superior anterolat-
eral aspect of the thigh.
I. After surgery and bracing, a patient can:
  1. Handle his toilet needs with minimal help.
  2. Facilitate transfer when his braces are locked at the knees
    and his legs used as a long lever to tilt him to the standing
    position.
J. The additional period of independent ambulation and therapeutic standing attained through these procedures may represent up to 20% of the life span of such patients. It can prove
of significant benefit to both them and their caretakers, as
maintenance of the upright posture has extended their ability

to attend to the tasks of daily living for a significant portion of
their lives.

III. Foot deformity (Fig 17–11). Even a minor degree of asymmetry in
a weight-bearing joint secondary to contracture can seriously interfere with balance and ambulation. Where possible, symmetric
posture should be maintained by bilateral foot surgery.

A. Foot drop (equinus):

1. Facioscapulohumeral dystrophy, secondary to weakness of
tibialis anticus, can be managed with an ankle-foot orthosis
that may be patellar weight bearing (Fig 17–12).

2. Dystrophia myotonica. Weak ankle dorsiflexion causes a
steppage type gait. Treat with an ankle-foot orthosis and
where quadriceps is weak; utilize floor reaction (built-in
equinus) feature.

3. Hereditary motor and sensory neuropathics usually do not
tolerate a plastic AFO well as the orthosis blocks the kinesthetic input required for balance. Because of distal sensory
and proprioceptive loss, such patients may shift their
weight at the ankles or knees in an attempt to "sense" the
supporting surface at more proximally placed joints, where
proprioception is intact. Ultimately, they require their

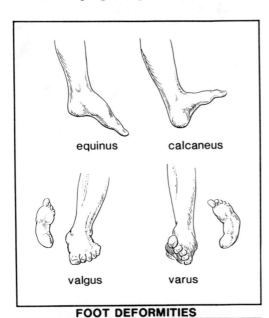

equinus   calcaneus

valgus   varus

FOOT DEFORMITIES

FIG 17–11.
Foot deformities.

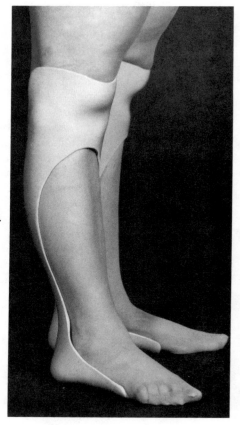

FIG 17–12.
Thermoplastic AFOs.

hands for balance, literally "elevating" the floor to hand level for proprioceptive input. Equinus in this class of disease is best managed with a light spring-loaded dorsiflexion assist orthosis. Posterior tibial transfer or (when fixed bony deformity is severe) osteotomy or tarsal arthrodesis can be performed.

4. DMD.
   a) Forefoot equinus is usually seen in children 5–10 years old and secondary to plantar fascia tightness. Best treated by plantar release.
   b) Hindfoot equinus is typically seen in patients 10 years of age or older, secondary to heel cord contracture. Treat with Achilles tenotomy (may add posterior tibial

release or transfer). Heel cord stretching should be continued after surgery as recurrence can occur where abnormal muscle does not lengthen as the bone grows.

(1) Percutaneous tenotomy is preferred, but when contracture of the posterior capsule of the ankle joint has occurred secondary to prolonged equinus, Z-plasty may be necessary to gain access to the posterior ankle for capsular release. Toe flexors may shorten with protracted equinus, and toe flexion may require stretching or release after Achilles tenotomy.

(2) Posterior tibial release or transfer can be performed by any of the standard operative methods, either to prevent anticipated or treat established soft tissue deformity.

(c) Equinocavovarus (Fig 17–13) ultimately occurs because of progressive selective weakening and asymmetric contracture of foot musculature. Once beyond the tibial-talar sagittal midline almost all dorsal and volar muscu-

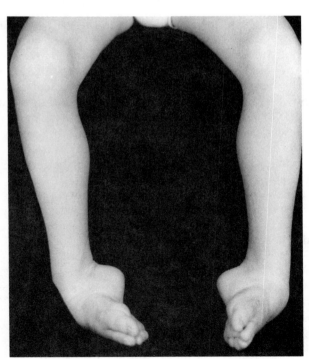

FIG 17–13.
Equinocavovarus.

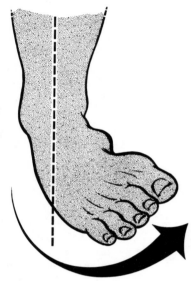

FIG 17–14.
Beyond sagittal plane, most foot and ankle
musculature furthers inversion.

lature, intrinsic and extrinsic, works to further inversion
(Fig 17–4).

(1) May temporarily respond to passive stretch and heel
control shoe inserts (e.g., UCB model).

(2) Early, before bony deformity has occurred, correction can be obtained by soft tissue release (heel cord,
posterior tibial) and bracing; heel cord lengthening
removes the stabilizing equinus force that hyperex-
tends and locks the knee during stance, so unless
the quadriceps is graded fair strength or better, the
knee must be braced.

(3) Later, with calcaneocavus bony deformity, soft tissue releases (tibialis posticus, plantar fascia) are augmented by percutaneous tarsal medullostomy of the
talar head and anterior portion of the calcaneus (Fig
17–15). Correction is obtained by manipulation of
the foot with collapse of the enucleated bones. A
short leg plaster is worn for three weeks followed by
an appropriate "best corrected position" AFO.

    (a) Tarsal fusion (triple arthrodesis) is contraindi-
cated because of the prolonged immobilization
required with this operation, which is interdic-

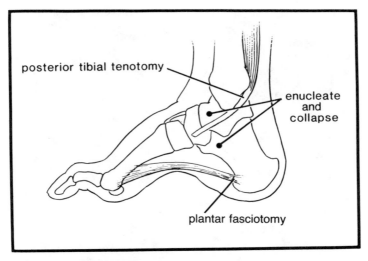

FIG 17–15.
Treatment of calcaneo-cavus deformity.

tory in the treatment of children with Duchenne muscular dystrophy.

(b) If the patient is wheelchair confined (Fig 17–16), where standing balance and ambulation are no longer feasible, a midtarsal dorsolateral closing wedge osteotomy (Fig 17–17) is the treatment of choice (osteoclasis or talectomy are alternate procedures). This may be indicated because deformity can become severe enough to prevent the use of ordinary footwear and lateral pressure decubiti can develop even in nonweight-bearing patients.

B. Miscellaneous.

1. Metatarsus adductus (Fig 17–18). This isolated deformity is sometimes seen in childhood polymyositis and can be treated with percutaneous proximal osteotomy of the metatarsals followed by casts and orthoses.

2. Forefoot inversion is occasionally found in polymyositis and responds to dorsolateral transfer of the tibialis anticus tendon or split tibialis anticus transfer. These procedures remove a deforming inversion force, creating an active dorsiflexor working in neutral or eversion.

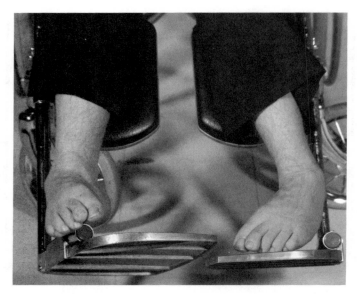

FIG 17–16.
Foot deformity in wheelchair-confined DMD.

3. Cavus occurs in Charcot-Marie-Tooth disease and Friedreich's ataxia (Fig 17–19). It is usually asymmetrical and
   worse on the side habitually relaxed while standing. Calcaneus deformity results from weakness of the triceps surae
   in the presence of strong ankle dorsiflexors. The relative
   muscle mass of plantar to dorsiflexors is in the ratio of four
   to one.

FIG 17–17.
Dorsolateral midtarsal wedge
resection.

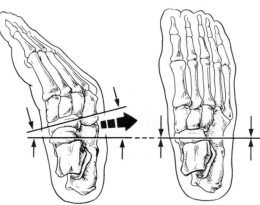

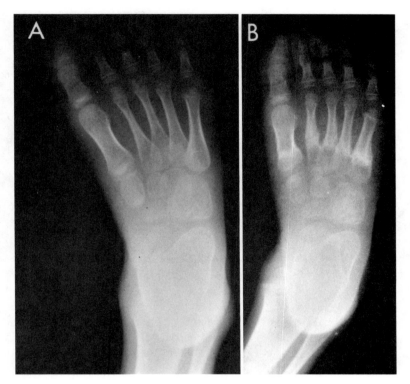

FIG 17–18.
A, metatarsus adductus—AP x-ray preop. **B,** metatarsus adductus—AP x-ray six weeks postop.

The relatively long lever arm of the ankle dorsiflexors as compared to triceps surae (in the presence of a paralyzed calf) can result in rapid progression of calcaneocavus deformity. In addition, there is dysfunction of the intrinsic foot muscles. If heel varus can be passively corrected when the heel is blocked up, throwing most of the weight onto the forefoot, correction of the forefoot alone (metatarsal osteotomy) should secondarily correct the hindfoot deformity. For fixed cavus with heel varus, the most popular corrective procedure is the triple arthrodesis, but this can result in a heavy awkward gait, and foot height may be decreased to the point where oxford shoes are difficult to fit because the malleoli impinge on the edge of the shoe counter. In any case, it should not be performed prior to

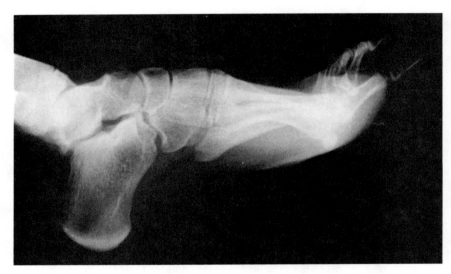

FIG 17–19.
Lateral x-ray, calcaneocavus foot.

age 10 because of the resulting shortening of the foot and
the potential for aseptic necrosis of the talus. Preferred is a
modified Dwyer (lateral closing wedge) calcaneal osteotomy
combined with the Mitchell (plantar fasciotomy with proximal displacement calcaneal osteotomy) procedure (Fig 17–
20). This operation effectively lenthens the heel, which
makes the fitting of a shoe (or a brace) easier. It can be
augmented by dorsal closing wedge proximal metatarsal
osteotomies (usually the first and second metatarsals) as indicated. Flexible cavus in the younger patient may respond
to plaster wedgings to stretch the heel into valgus (5 degrees) and correct forefoot pronation. This can be followed
by naviculocuneiform fusion. Extensor hallucis longus
transplantation to the first metatarsal head with metatarsal
phalangeal capsulotomy and interphalangeal fusion of the
great toe may be necessary to correct cock-up deformity of
this digit.
4. Hammertoes are seen in HSMN and allied conditions, and
   are best treated by waist resection of the proximal pha-
   langes or extensor tenotomy coupled with dorsal capsulotomy of the involved metatarsal-phalangeal joints and
   proximal interphalangeal fusion.

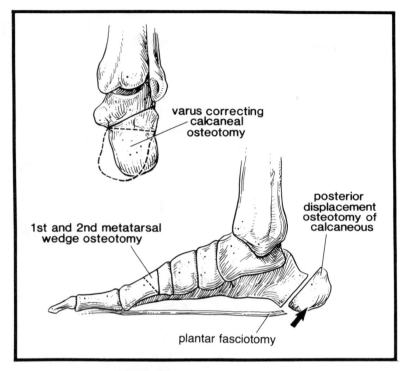

FIG 17–20.
Surgical correction of cavovarus foot.

5. Flail (noncontracted) lower extremities (in SMA). The reciprocation-gait orthosis (a light weight-bracing system providing structural support to the trunk and legs while allowing hip joint motion for ambulation through a cable coupling device) has proved effective in selected cases (Fig 17–21).
6. Pes valgus is seen in ambulatory SMA because of generalized hypotonia. It is aggravated by peroneal tendon contracture with weak triceps surae muscle group. Treat by transferring peroneus longus and brevis to the os calcis. An AFO is necessary after surgery.
7. Pes arcuatum (elevation of the lateral arch) found in neuromuscular disease (e.g., Friedreich's ataxia) may require intrinsic foot release.
8. Talipes equinovarus (in neonatal dystrophia myotonica) requires serial cast correction from birth and tends to recur if

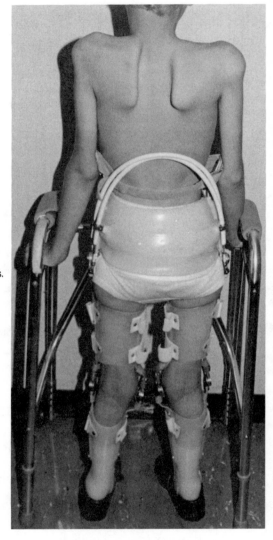

FIG 17–21.
Reciprocation-gait orthosis.

not held by bivalved casts or AFOs. Such feet may need
extensive soft tissue releases and/or triple arthrodesis at
skeletal maturity to maintain correction. Valgus deformity
of the interphalangeal joint of the hallux may require surgical correction (fusion).

IV. Knee problems.
  A. Chondromalacia patellae is found in patients unable to extend their knees because of flexion contracture. Pain is usually not severe enough to require treatment beyond symptomatic care.
  B. Genu recurvatum is seen in diseases where lower extremity weakness is severe and contracture minimal. If quadriceps strength is adequate, knee position and stance can be controlled by an AFO where ankle motion is locked in neutral or slight dorsiflexion, thus preventing back knee.
  C. Knee weakness with patterning. Though most patients with

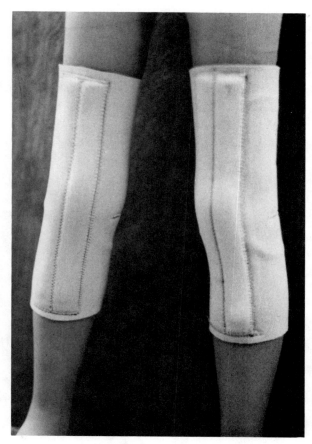

FIG 17–22.
Quadriceps assist orthoses.

Duchenne muscular dystrophy walk in external rotation, some develop hip joint valgus and anteversion with subsequent internal rotation of the lower extremities. Although hip extensors (gluteus maximus) and knee extensors (quadriceps) are weak and lack of fixed ankle equinus can prevent the floor-reaction response necessary for passive knee extension, patients such as this are able to walk using residual strength in hip adductor and hamstring muscles. In such cases, the use of quadriceps assist orthoses (neoprene knee sleeves reinforced anteriorly by clockspring steel stays wound to assist knee extension) can often augment quadriceps strength just enough to keep the patient upright and maintain ambulation (Fig 17–22).

V. Hip problems.
   A. Congenital dislocation of the hip(s) is frequently seen in the morphologically specific myopathies, particularly central core disease. Treatment is along standard lines, but open reduction with augmented surgery to assure stability and maintain reduction may be necessary.

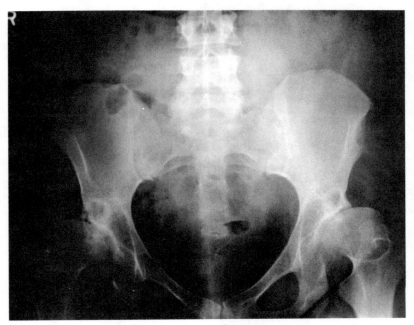

FIG 17–23.
Neurotrophic arthropathic hips in CMT.

B. In Charcot-Marie-Tooth disease, the hips are frequently incongruous, may require surgical reconstruction, and can develop degenerative (neurotrophic-arthropathic) changes (Fig 17–23).

In summary, a judicious choice among the relatively simple surgical procedures outlined above, followed by immediate postoperative mobilization, can often prolong walking. As the patient's ability to ambulate diminishes, one must determine whether this is the result of weakness, contracture, or both. The earlier surgery is done, the better the result. Except for operations prophylactically performed (e.g., early transfer of posterior tibial muscle), the indications for lower extremity surgery are contractures sufficient to threaten the upright posture. The conditions for such procedures are enough strength to motivate braced extremities postoperatively and, of course, cardiorespiratory reserves adequate to survive the operation.

BIBLIOGRAPHY

Armstrong RM, Koeningsberger R, Mellinger J, et al: Central core disease with congenital hip dislocation. *Neurology* 1975; 21:369–376.

Bonsett CA: Prophylactic bracing in pseudohypertrophic muscular dystrophy (preliminary report). Part I, Patient Experience, and Part II, The Brace. *Indiana Med* 1975; 68:(181):185–187.

Bowker JH, Halpin PJ: Factors determining success in reambulation of the child with progressive muscular dystrophy. *Orthop Clin North Am* 1978; 9:431–436.

Coleman SS, Chesnut WJ: A simple test for hind foot flexibility in the cavovarus foot. *Clin Orthop* 1977; 123:60–62.

Drennan J: *Orthopedic Management of Neuromuscular Disorders*. Philadelphia, JB Lippincott, Co, 1983.

Eyring EJ, Johnson EW, Burnett CPT: Surgery in muscular dystrophy. *JAMA* 1972; 222:1056–1057.

Falewski de Leon G: Maintenance of mobility. *Isr J Med Sci* 1977; 13:177–182.

Gucker T, III: The orthopedic management of progressive muscular dystrophy. *J Phys Ther* 1964; 44:228–243.

Heckmatt JZ, et al: Prolongation of walking in Duchenne muscular dystrophy with lightweight orthoses: Review of 57 cases. *Dev Med Child Neurol* 1985; 27:149–154.

Hsu JD: Management of foot deformity in Duchenne's pseudohypertrophic muscular dystrophy. *Orthop Clin North Am* 1976; 7:979–984.

Hyde SA, et al: Prolongation of ambulation in Duchenne muscular dystrophy by appropriate orthoses. *Physiotherapy* 1982; 68:105–108.

Kaneda RR: Becker's muscular dystrophy: Orthopedic implications. *J Am Osteopath Assoc* 1980; 79:332–335.

Lehmann JF: Biomechanics of ankle-foot orthoses: Prescription and design. *Arch Phys Med Rehabil* 1979; 60:200–207.

McElvenny RT, Caldwell GD: A new operation for correction of cavus foot: Fusion of first metatarsocuneiform navicular joints. *Clin Orthop* 1958; 11: 85–92.

Miller J: Management of muscular dystrophy *J Bone Joint Surg* 1967; 49A: 1205–1211.

Nuzzo RM: Dynamic bracing: Elastics for patients with cerebral palsy, muscular dystrophy, and myelodysplasia. *Clin Orthop* 1980; 148:263–273.

Ramsey PL, Hensinger RN: Congenital dislocation of the hip associated with central core disease. *J Bone Joint Surg* 1975; 57A:648–651.

Ray S, Bowen JR, Marks HG: Foot deformity in myotonic dystrophy. *Foot Ankle* 1984; 5:125–130.

Ray S, Bowen JR, Marks HG: Congenital dislocation of the hip and hip dysplasia in Charcot-Marie-Tooth disease. *Contemp Orthop* 1985; 11:19–23.

Reinherz R, Mann I: Lower extremity involvement in Duchenne muscular dystrophy. *J Am Podiatr Assoc* 1977; 67:796–801.

Rochelle J Bowen JR, Ray S: Pediatric foot deformities in progressive neuromuscular disease. *Contemp Orthop* 1984; 8:41–50.

Roy I, Gibson DA: Pseudohypertrophic muscular dystrophy and its surgical management: Review of 30 patients. *Can J Surg* 1970; 13:13–21.

Samilson RL: Calcaneocavus feet: A plan of management in children. *Orthop Rev* 1981; 10:121–124.

Siegel IM: Equinocavovarus in muscular dystrophy: Treatment by percutaneous tarsal medullostomy and soft tissue release. *Isr J Med Sci* 1977; 13:189–191.

Siegel IM: Plastic-molded knee-ankle-foot orthoses in the treatment of Duchenne muscular dystrophy. *Arch Phys Med Rehabil* 1975; 56:322.

Siegel IM, Miller JE, Ray RD: Subcutaneous lower limb tenotomy in the treatment of pseudohypertrophic muscular dystrophy. *J Bone Joint Surg* 1968; 50A:1437–1443.

Siegel IM: Equinocavovarus in muscular dystrophy. *Arch Surg* 1972; 104: 644–646.

Siegel IM, Silverman O: Double cylinder plastic orthosis in the treatment of Duchenne muscular dystrophy. *Phys Ther* 1981; 15:1290–1291.

Siegel IM: Diagnosis, management and orthopaedic treatment of muscular dystrophy: Instructional course lectures. *Am Acad Orthop Surg* 1981; 30:3–35.

Silver RL, De La Garza J, Rang M: The myth of muscle balance *J Bone Joint Surg* 1985; 67B: 432–437.

Spencer GE, Jr: Orthopaedic care of progressive muscular dystrophy. *J Bone Joint Surg* 1967; 49A:1201–1204.

Spencer GE, Jr, Vignos JP, Jr: Bracing for ambulation in childhood progressive muscular dystrophy. *J Bone Joint Surg* 1962; 44A:234–242.

Spencer GE, Jr: Orthopaedic considerations in the management of muscular dystrophy, in Ahstrom J (ed): *Recent Advances in Orthopedics*. Baltimore, Williams & Wilkins Co, 1973, pp 279–293.

Vignos PJ, Jr, Archibald KC: Maintenance of ambulation in childhood muscular dystrophy. *J Chronic Dis* 1960; 12:273–290.

Vignos PJ, Jr, Wagner MB, Kaplan JS, et al: Predicting the success of reambulation in patients with Duchenne muscular dystrophy. *J Bone Joint Surg* 1983; 65A:719–728.

Ziter FA, Allsop KG: Comprehensive treatment of childhood muscular dystrophy. *Rocky Mtn Med J* 1975; 72:329–333.

18

Treatment: Upper Extremities

"The practice of medicine is an art based on a science."
Sir William Osler (1849–1919)
"The lesser the indication, the greater the complication."
Hawkins Law for Surgeons

I. Hand.
  A. For optional grasp function, the hand must open, close, and open again. Hand function can be analyzed as follows:
    1. Precision grip (Fig 18–1,A).
      a) Thumb-tip, index, and middle fingers.
      b) Thumb-pulp, index, and middle fingers (three joint chuck).
    2. Transition grip.
      a) Lateral prehension—key grip.
      b) "Screwdriver" grip.
    3. Power grasp (Fig 18–1,B).
      a) Hook.
      b) Sphere.
      c) Small cylinder.
      d) Large cylinder.
  B. Hand disability.
    1. Weakness is not problematic in DMD until late in the dis-

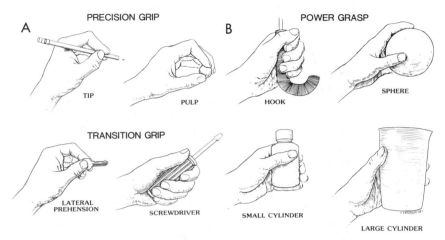

PRECISION GRIP

A

TIP

PULP

POWER GRASP

B

HOOK

SPHERE

TRANSITION GRIP

LATERAL PREHENSION

SCREWDRIVER

SMALL CYLINDER

LARGE CYLINDER

FIG 18–1.
Hand function patterns.

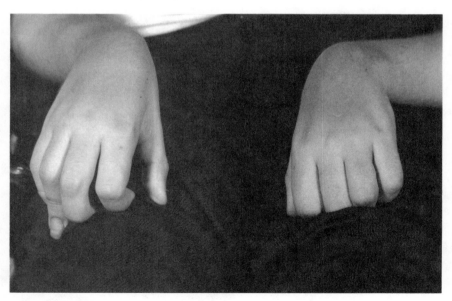

FIG 18–2.
Wrist flexion: ulnar deviation and finger flexion deformity in wheelchair-confined DMD.

ease, and then is usually best treated with adaptive equipment. (e.g., balanced forearm orthosis). When a child is wheelchair confined, he tends to hold his elbows in flexion, and gravity pulls the wrists into ulnar deviation and flexion (Fig 18–2). Resulting wrist contracture should be passively stretched and splinted in a functional position.

2. Weakness of thumb opposition found in dystrophia myotonica, distal myopathy, and certain neuropathies can be treated with a light plastic orthosis that firmly fixes the thumb as a post to stabilize opposition pinch.

3. Hand weakness, though not prominent in neuronal Charcot-Marie-Tooth disease, is seen in its hypertrophic counterpart, and surgery (tendon-transfers, opponensplasty) to compensate for median and/or ulnar motor loss with intrinsic hand deformity, can be helpful in older patients. Occasionally, thenar metacarpaltrapezium subluxation (Fig 18–3) or dislocation will render the thumb unstable, requiring fixation by splintage or arthrodesis.

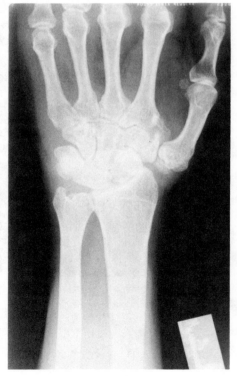

FIG 18–3.
HMSN 1: metacarpal-trapezium subluxation.

4. Tendon transfer to increase wrist and/or finger function of the upper extremity may be indicated in selected patients with slowly progressive muscular atrophy (e.g., segmental muscular atrophy of adolescence).

II. Elbow.

A. Generally, the upper extremities develop contractures less frequently and less severely than do the lower because even in the wheelchair, they maintain a range of motion during activities while the legs remain still.

1. Mild elbow flexion contracture can be found in ambulatory DMD as these patients "wing" their arms for balance while walking. Elbow flexion contracture with forearm pronation and wrist flexion-ulnar deviation occurs in wheelchair-confined DMD patients (Fig 18–4). This is the position in

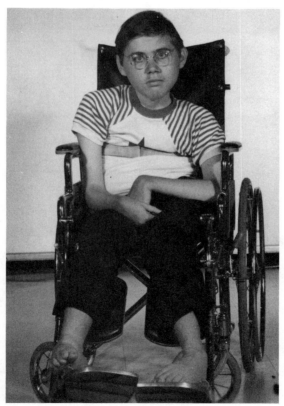

FIG 18–4.
Elbow flexion with forearm pronation deformity in wheelchair-confined DMD.

which the arm is held most of the time for function. Elbow flexion contracture greater than 60 degrees severely interferes with functional activities, but some flexion contracture (15 degrees) may prove adaptive in assisting the initiation of movement for performing motor tasks in the face of severe forearm weakness.

2. Wheelchair-confined patients with neuromuscular disease (particularly peripheral neuropathies) are predisposed to compression neuropathy. Most commonly seen is ulnar neuritis secondary to wheelchair arm pressure on the elbow and forearm. In the normal elbow, the force for lifting the forearm is supplied by the biceps with a short (third degree) lever distance from the biceps insertion to the fulcrum at the olecranon. With loss of biceps function, the forearm is "lifted" by applying downward force to tilt the elbow through a fulcrum supplied in the mid to distal forearm by

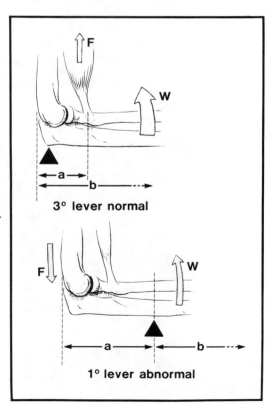

FIG 18–5.
Forces about the elbow joint.

the armrests of the chair (Fig 18–5). This (first degree) lever arm is kept long to minimize the force necessary to move the member, and pressure can be repeatedly imposed upon the ulnar nerve.

III. Shoulder.

    A. In DMD or LGD, the shoulders may contract in internal rotation. This is because these patients find it necessary to flex the elbow, hooking the thumbs over the side pockets of their slacks or through a belt loop (internally rotating the shoulder and pronating the wrist), thus unloading the upper extremities and using them to balance, much as a tightrope walker utilizes a pole (Fig 18–6). This position is necessary for standing and walking stability and should not be discouraged.

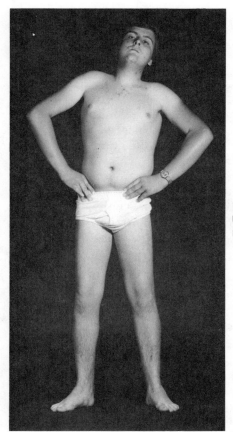

FIG 18–6.
Using the upper extremities for balance (LGD).

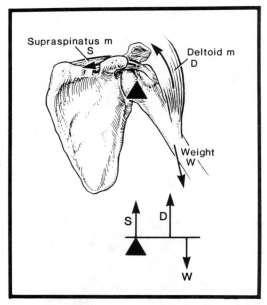

FIG 18–7.
The shoulder is a 3rd-degree lever.

Later, shoulder weakness in the wheelchair-confined patient is best managed with forearm orthoses so balanced to allow the arms to move across rather than against the gravity field, thus assisting TDL (eating, writing, etc).

B. In FSH, shoulder stabilizer weakness can early on significantly interfere with upper extremity function, especially with such tasks as eating and overhead dressing. The shoulder is a third degree lever system, sacrificing strength for range of motion (Fig 18–7). The scapula must be fixed to the posterior chest

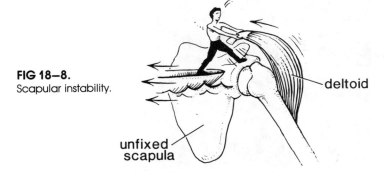

FIG 18–8.
Scapular instability.

wall to allow the deltoid its mechanical advantage in rotating the humeral head in the glenoid. The first 30 degrees of shoulder abduction is at the glenohumeral joint. After this, abduction occurs at the glenohumeral and scapulothoracic joints in a 2-to-1 ratio. With inadequate scapular stability, any attempt to use the deltoid for abduction is like trying to step to a dock from an untethered boat (Fig 18–8). In selected cases with preserved deltoid function (approximately 50% of all FSH) the following surgical procedures are available for scapular stabilization:

1. Screw fixation of scapula to posterior ribs.
2. Fusion through bone graft between posterior ribs and deep scapular surface, augmented by wire-loop fixation of scapula to ribs (Fig 18–9).
3. Scapular fixation, either interscapular or to posterior ribs, through fascial ties.

C. After scapular fixation, by whatever means, patients no longer require a "thrown" movement to elevate the arm. The scapula should not be fixed with its vertebral border more than 20 de-

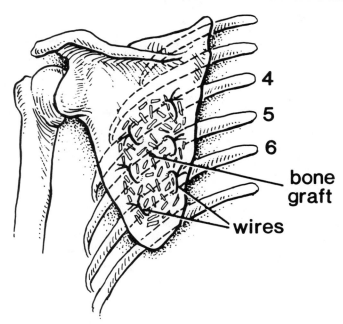

4
5
6
bone graft
wires

FIG 18–9.
Scapulothoracic fusion using wire and bone graft.

grees from the vertical. It is necessary to allow at least one upper extremity the freedom to attend to toileting tasks. Immobilizing three or four ribs decreases chest compliance and results in a 10%–20% decrease in vital capacity of the involved lung.

BIBLIOGRAPHY

Bunch WH: Scapulo-thoracic fusion for shoulder stabilization in muscular dystrophy. *Minn Med* 1973; 56:391–394.
Copeland SA, Howard RC: Thoracoscapular fusion for facioscapulohumeral dystrophy. *J Bone Joint Surg* 1978; 60B:547–551.
Drennan J: *Orthopedic Management of Neuromuscular Disorders.* Philadelphia, JB Lippincott, Co, 1983.
Ketenjian AY: Muscular dystrophy: Diagnosis and treatment. *Orthop Clin North Am* 1978; 9:25–42.
Siegel IM: Early signs of Landouzy-Dejerine disease: Wrist and finger weakness. *JAMA* 1972; 221:302.
Sinaki M, Wood MB, Mulder DW: Rehabilitative operation for motor neuron disease: Tendon transfer for segmental muscular atrophy of the upper extremities. *Mayo Clin Proc* 1984; 59:338–342.
Spira E: The treatment of dropped shoulder. *J Bone Joint Surg* 1948; 30A: 229–233.
Walton JN (ed): *Disorders of Voluntary Muscles,* ed 4. New York, Churchill Livingstone, Inc, 1981.

19

Scoliosis

"Good advice is no better than bad advice unless taken at the right time."

Danish proverb

Scoliosis, occurring in many different neuromuscular diseases affecting children, now comprises 15%–20% of all spinal deformity treated by the orthopedic surgeon.

I. Occurrence.
   A. Neuropathic disorders, such as poliomyelitis, cerebral palsy (25%), idiopathic relapsing polyneuropathy, chronic infantile and juvenile spinal muscular atrophy (95%), the various spinal cerebellar ataxias (85%), myelomeningocele (70%), familial dysautonomia, and Charcot-Marie-Tooth disease (58%).
   B. Myopathies, such as Duchenne muscular dystrophy (80%), childhood facioscapulohumeral dystrophy, Becker's dystrophy, the childhood form of dystrophia myotonica, postinfantile acid-maltase deficiency.
   C. Other neuromuscular conditions of as yet uncertain etiology, such as nemaline rod disease, central core disease, Prader-Willi syndrome, and oculocraniosomatic neuromuscular disease with "ragged red" fibers.

    D. It is also believed that children with "idiopathic" scoliosis, without evidence of developmental and acquired focal lesions of the spine and spinal cord, may suffer from a subclinical neuromuscular condition, asymmetrically affecting the paraspinal musculature, causing coronal spinal deformity.

  II. Etiologic factors in neuromuscular scoliosis include:*
    A. Brain or spinal cord lesion.
    B. Paralysis of the limb girdle or trunk muscles.
    C. Progressive weakness, muscle imbalance, disuse atrophy.
    D. Pelvic obliquity.
    E. The effects of growth.

 III. Differences between idiopathic and neuromuscular scoliosis:
    A. Deformity and disease are often progressive in neuromuscular scoliosis.
    B. Curve patterns develop earlier and are more likely to progress beyond skeletal maturity and through life in neuromuscular scoliosis.
    C. Neuromuscular disease may produce a deformity involving not only the spine, but also the pelvis, hips, and legs.
    D. Multisystem involvement can occur in the disease process.
    E. Regarding the treatment of scoliosis in neuromuscular disease, bone stock is usually quantitatively and qualitatively poor, there is less tolerance for orthotic devices, and, with spinal fusion, the rate of pseudarthrosis is high.

 IV. Paralytic scoliosis in muscular dystrophy.
    A. One of the most serious complications of the muscular dystrophies. Forced vital capacity is decreased by 4% for each 10 degrees of thoracic scoliosis (as well as by the same amount for each year of age after onset of the curve). This diminution in pulmonary function is not recoverable after surgical curve correction.
    B. Occurs with advancing disability determined by the type of dystrophy with progress related to severity of the disease.
      1. Limb-girdle dystrophy usually occurs at or near the time when spinal growth is completed, weakness is often symmetric, and progression slow. Although a functional spinal

---

*Spinal stability is not only related to the vertebral bony structures but also to the status of the intervertebral discs, joint capsules, facet joints, ligaments of the spinal column, and its muscular support. Proprioception and spinal cord reflexes are vital in maintaining spinal equilibrium. The pelvis must be level and the neck, back, and shoulder muscles symmetrically intact in order to preserve upright posture of the spine. Spinal stability is directly related to the end support of the spinal axis and inversely proportional to the flexibility of the vertebral column and the square of its length.

curve is occasionally seen, patients with LGD ambulate into their second or third decade, and structural scoliosis is an uncommon finding.

2. Progressive scoliosis is often seen in childhood dystrophia myotonica, the childhood type of FSH (Fig 19–1), and the Becker form of muscular dystrophy. In these conditions, asymmetry of muscle weakness can cause scoliosis while the patient is yet ambulatory.

3. DMD-paraspinal weakness is symmetric (Fig 19–2), and scoliosis occurs rarely and then usually with pelvic or infra-pelvic obliquity secondary to uncorrected lower extremity contracture. Pelvic tilt or asymmetric arm positioning can also unbalance the torso and contort the spine (Fig 19–3

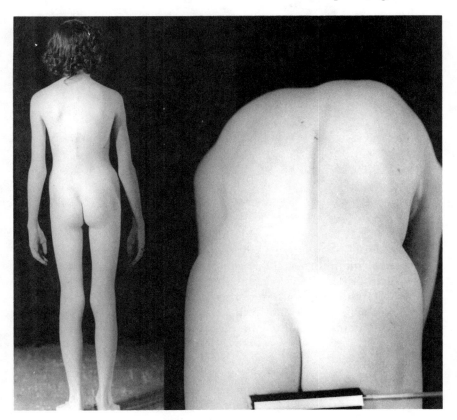

FIG 19–1.
Scoliosis in childhood FSH.

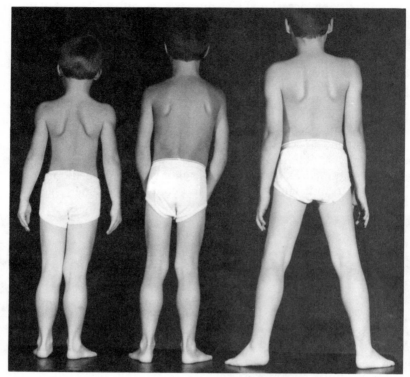

FIG 19–2.
Three brothers with DMD. Symmetric paraspinal weakness. No scoliosis.

and 19–4). Patients who are standing and/or walking "lordose" their spines, shifting the center of gravity forward to maintain torso-pelvic balance. This locks the lumbar and lumbosacral facets, inhibiting lateral deformity. Therapeutic standing is an important part of the prophylactic treatment of spinal deformity in this class of patient. Alternating symmetrical and asymmetrical spinal stretching exercise is provided by body weight shifting over the supporting leg during the stance phase of gait. This is why such children often find crutches or a cane an encumbrance rather than an aid. These appliances prevent the upper extremity positioning required for balance. Severe caution should be exercised when attempting to straighten and/or stabilize the spine of a walking DMD patient, either surgically or orthot-

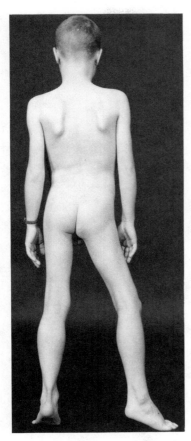

FIG 19–3.
Scoliosis from pelvic tilt in DMD.

ically. Fixing the spine to the pelvis may prevent ambulation, and any spinal rigidity (particularly at the eighth thoracic level, the nodal point for spinal axis rotation) can inhibit ambulation. Once wheelchair-bound, patients with DMD tend to lean to the nondominant side, freeing the dominant upper extremity for functional use. Overuse of the dominant extremity can unbalance the unsupported growing spine and result in scoliosis with the major convexity toward the dominant side. Spinal extension is often lost, particularly when the arms weaken to where they can no longer propel the chair and the patient leans forward, using the body to assist movement. Loss of normal lordosis or kyphosis makes the spine more vulnerable for scoliotic

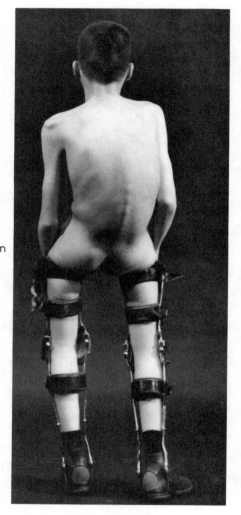

FIG 19—4.
DMD. Pelvic tilt and kyphoscoliosis in braces.

deformity. Because spinal deformity in postambulatory patients is almost inevitable, ambulation should be prolonged as long as possible through contracture release and lower extremity bracing. Patients wheelchair confined after completion of vertebral growth, where agonist-antagonist paraspinal muscle groups have atrophied to the same level of weakness, stand a better chance of avoiding spinal deformity in the wheelchair. Additionally, when a patient can no longer independently turn in bed, a dorsal spinal curvature tends to develop, convex to the side on which he lies.

Although approximately one-third of paralytic curves in DMD are minimally unstable, scoliosis (commonly thoracolumbar-kyphotic with unstable axial rotation) may progress rapidly, especially during the adolescent growth spurt. These curves are typically low and associated with pelvic tilt. After onset they progress at about 2.2 degrees to 2.6 degrees per month until age 13 when they undergo rapid decompensation. There is loss of normal coupled segmental spinal motion in these patients, leading to severe spinal deformity and biplanar imbalance. Double curves modulate into lumbar and thoracolumbar curves. Pelvic tilt increases. Such curves pose major functional and cosmetic problems, including:

a) The need to use the upper limbs for support because of impaired sitting balance.
b) Loss of bimanual function.
c) Cardiopulmonary compromise.
d) Impoverished body image.
e) Occasionally pain, accompanying advancing deformity.
f) Loss of functional head position.
g) Ischial decubiti (rarely).

V. Treatment.
A. Orthoses are indicated for short-term daytime use to maintain upright sitting balance in curves less than 30 degrees or following spinal fusion; also, for long-term sitting support where spinal fusion is medically contraindicated (e.g., where vital capacity is essentially the same as tidal volume).
1. A thoracic orthosis providing three-point fixation, fitted to hold the lumbar spine in lordosis and limiting lateral spinal mobility, can produce a rigid extended spine (flexible lordosis has not proven protective), slowing the development of scoliosis (Fig 19–5). However, such an appliance may weaken paraspinal musculature, fail to control the progress of curvature, and at times compromise rib compliance, decreasing pulmonary function.
2. The Milwaukee brace has not proven useful in the treatment of neuromuscular scoliosis because this is a dynamic appliance requiring enough residual muscle strength for the patient to move in the brace.
3. The thoracic suspension orthosis has been helpful in sus-

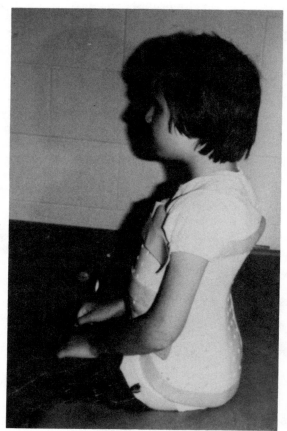

FIG 19–5.
TLSO exaggerating lumbar lordosis.

pending patients to avoid ischial pressure while treating decubitus ulcers in those with severe respiratory problems and in curves too advanced to lend themselves to more conventional orthotic treatment.

4. Orthoses can be constructed of Silastic, Orthoplast, isoprene, polyethylene, polypropylene, or Subortholene. A firm level pelvic seat (if the pelvis is stabilized, the critical vertical load necessary to produce lateral spinal deformity must be doubled) should be provided when wheelchair confinement is inevitable, before the onset of spinal curvature. At this time the spine is flaccid and responds to the exoskeletal thoracopelvic distribution forces such a jacket provides. Spinal alignment is obtained by fitting the TLSO

with the patient in cervical traction, supporting the abdomen, elevating the ribs from a contoured pelvic foundation and (utilizing residual neck extension strength) forcing the shoulders back, exaggerating lumbar lordosis and locking the lumbar and lumbosacral facet joints, to inhibit lateral spinal bending. With correction of abdominal ptosis, the diaphragm has increased freedom of movement. It has been reported that spinal support inhibiting scoliosis helps maintain lung compliance and enhances vital capacity in DMD.

5. The wheelchair is an orthosis, and specialized wheelchair seating may achieve spinal containment. The Toronto spinal support system, the Chicago wheelchair insert (Fig 19–6), as well as a variety of vacuum molded seating systems are designed to mold the spine into lordosis and provide lateral stability (Fig 19–7). It is essential that the spine be extended in such an apparatus, and this usually requires at least 15 degrees of posterior tilt in the adapted wheelchair. It is emphasized that these systems will seldom prevent scoliosis. Rather, they may delay the development of spinal deformity and reduce its rate of progression by about 50%. At the same time, they provide comfortable, functional seating.

6. Limitations to the use of these conservative methods include:
   a) Rapidly progressive curves beyond 45 degrees.
   b) Unbalanced curves.
   c) Cephalad extension of the curve above T6.
   d) Obesity.
   e) Pelvic tilt while seated.
   f) Loss of head control.
   g) Noncompliance.

B. Surgery.
   1. Indications. In the wheelchair-confined DMD patient or the ambulating childhood dystrophia myotonica, Becker's dystrophy, or childhood facioscapulohumeral dystrophy. In spinal muscular atrophy as well as Friedreich's ataxia, Charcot-Marie-Tooth disease, and familial dysautonomia. Finally, in selected cases of a variety of neuromuscular diseases requiring spinal stabilization.
   2. Conditions necessary for surgery.
      a) An unstable curve of 35–40 degrees.

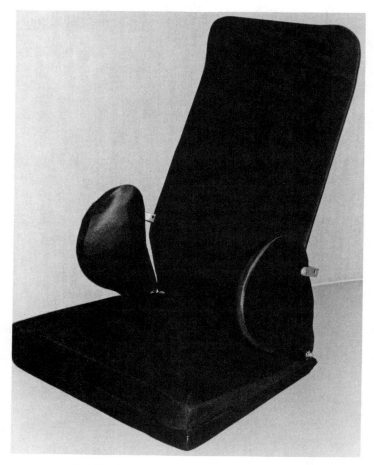

FIG 19–6.
Wheelchair insert for holding spine in extension.

b) Vital capacity within 35%–40% of predicted normal.
c) Ability to cough with an adequate forced expiratory volume.
d) Sufficient P_{O_2} (also, P_{CO_2} above 40 mm Hg indicates hypoventilation).
e) In patients yet ambulatory, an extensive spinal fusion to the pelvis may remove compensating mechanisms required for balanced ambulation (hyperlordosis to compensate for weak hip extensor muscles, maintaining the

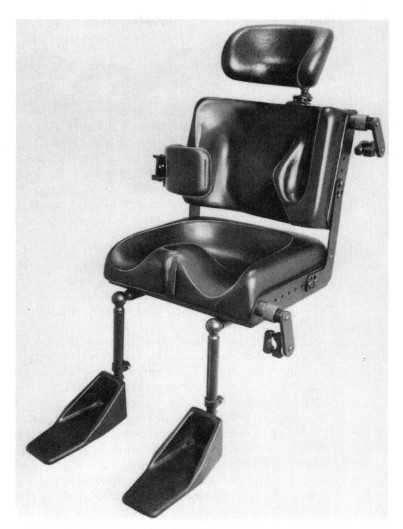

FIG 19–7.
Vacuum-molded seating system providing lordosis and lateral stability.

center of gravity within the base of support) and demote a walker to a permanent sitter.

  f) With curves great enough to present a high risk for neurological complications when straightened and those in the cervicothoracic region, as well as where pulmonary function requires improvement to permit surgery, preoperative spinal traction may be indicated.

3. Intraoperative considerations.
   a) Close monitoring of arterial blood gases, CVP, cardiac output, and urine output.
   b) Intraoperative monitoring of spinal cord function by somatosensory evoked potentials and/or wakeup test.
   c) Meticulous surgery to accomplish rigid arthrodesis and a balanced spine over a level pelvis.
   d) Blood transfusions (usually numerous since, in patients with DMD, the weakened fibrotic muscle mass does not contract well to aid vessel constriction).
   e) Hemodilution, hypotensive anesthesia, and autogenous blood transfusions or RBC saving techniques as available and indicated.

4. Postoperative care.
   a) Correcting a thoracic kyphosis can significantly increase the "dead space" along which air must be moved, and reduce pulmonary function by as much as 20% by restricting chest wall compliance. This may require (permanent) tracheostomy.
   b) Because of poor pulmonary reserve, patients with neuromuscular disease undergoing spinal surgery may suffer an absolute loss of vital capacity for several weeks after operation. This is related to overstretching of intercostal muscles on the convex side of the curve, with relaxation on the concave side, overexpansion of the convex, with compression of the concave lung, decreased reserve in the accessory muscles of respiration, and postoperative pain. The prolonged work of postoperative breathing is exhausting for these patients, and intensive pulmonary support (e.g., inhalation therapy and breathing exercises) during this time is vital. When prolonged ventilatory assistance is necessary, nasotracheal intubation is preferable to tracheostomy.
   c) Vital capacity and arterial oxygen level decrease where cast immobilization is necessary after surgery. It is therefore best to provide rigid spinal fixation, obviating the need for casts or braces postoperatively and permitting long-term sitting stability.
   d) In the early postoperative period, rehabilitation includes daily range of motion exercises to prevent contracture,

resistance exercises to maintain muscle strength, and later, appropriate training in body mechanics and transfer techniques.

e) Patients must be monitored closely, utilizing radiologic techniques such as tomography, CT, and bone scanning to detect pseudarthrosis.

5. Surgical techniques. With appropriate indications (improving ambulatory independence in selected patients or establishing independent sitting balance in the wheelchair-confined dystrophic or SMA with progressive spinal curvature unresponsive to external containment) and conditions (respiratory parameters adequate to survive surgery), operative spinal stabilization can be obtained through the following methods:

a) Harrington compression-distraction instrumentation (Fig 19–8), sometimes secured with wire to the spine at critical points.

b) L-rod segmental spinal stabilization of Luque. With this technique the rods can be contoured to secure a measure of kyphosis for head balance. Two rods can be used, or a single rod bent to the shape of two L-shaped

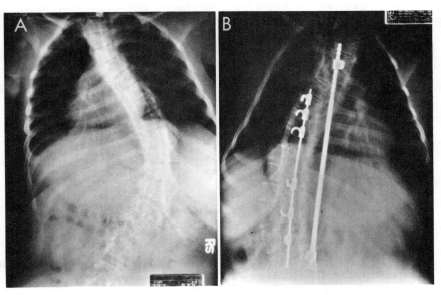

FIG 19–8.
A, scoliosis, preop. **B,** Harrington instrumentation.

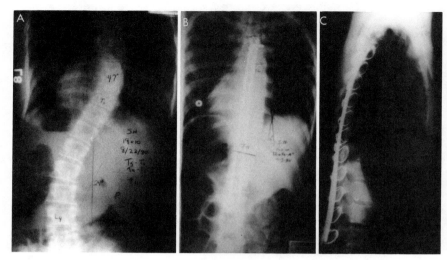

FIG 19–9.
A, scoliosis, preop. **B** and **C,** segmental (Luque) spinal stabilization.

rods joined at the top. This prevents translation of one
side with respect to the other. The operation has been
performed with and without accompanying bony fusion,
(laminar decortication and facet joint excision) and can
be augmented with methylmethacrylate bone cement, allowing early postoperative mobilization without the ne-
cessity for casting or bracing (Fig 19–9).

   c) A Moe subcutaneous rod can be used in the skeletally
   immature patient, thus delaying the inevitable long
   spinal fusion.

   d) Anterior fusion. The Dwyer cable technique is seldom
   indicated and then always supplemented with a posterior fusion.

   Stabilization of the spine (usually to the pelvis and extending several levels above the horizontal cephalad vertebra) improves body image, enhances cardiorespiratory function, obviates discomfort, frees the
upper extremities from a supportive role for more functional use, and
facilitates transfer. Obtaining spinal stability with the head in the midline through the correction of pelvic obliquity allows the patient both
improved cosmesis and increased function.

   Table 19–1 summarizes the surgical management of muscular dystrophy.

TABLE 19–1.
Surgical Management of Muscular Dystrophy

I. Lower Extremity
  A. "Prophylactic" (under 7 years)
    1. Posterior tibial transfer
    2. Tensor fasciae latae release
  B. Early (7 to 9 years)
    1. Heel cord or tensor fasciae latae release
      a) Quadriceps must be rated fair or better
      b) Fit floor-reaction orthosis
  C. Middle (9 to 12 years)
    1. Triple release (hip flexors, tensor fasciae latae, heel cords)
      a) Fit KAFO
    2. Posterior tibial ransfer or release
  D. Late (over 12 years)
    1. Tarsal medullostomy
      a) Posterior tibial release
      b) Plantar fasciotomy
  E. Foot deformity
    1. Forefoot equinus
      a) Plantar release—AFO
    2. Hindfoot equinus
      a) Achilles tenotomy
      b) Posterior tibial transfer
      c) Floor-reaction AFO
    3. Equinocavovarus
      a) Tarsal medullostomy
      b) Posterior tibial release
      c) Plantar fasciotomy
      d) Talectomy (rarely)
    4. Metatarsus adductus
      a) Percutaneous metatarsal osteotomies
    5. Forefoot inversion
      a) Tibialis anticus transfer
    6. Cavus
      a) Calcaneal osteotomy—plantar fasciotomy
      b) Metatarsal osteotomy
      c) Triple arthrodesis (on rare occasion)
    7. Claw toes
      a) Soft tissue release
      b) Phalangeal resection
      c) Interphalangeal fusion
  F. Hip dislocation (in "congenital" myopathies)
    1. Open reduction accompanied by appropriate acetabular or proximal
      femoral osteotomies and/or tendon transfer as indicated
II. Upper Extremity
  A. Median and/or ulnar loss in Charcot-Marie-Tooth
    1. Appropriate tendon transfers
  B. Shoulder weakness in FSH
    1. Scapular stabilization   *continued.*

Table 19–1.—Continued

III. Scoliosis
  A. Spinal fusion
    1. In ambulatory FSH and Becker's dystrophy, where indicated
    2. In wheelchair-bound DMD and SMA, when necessary

BIBLIOGRAPHY

Bernhang AM, Rosen H, Leivy D: Internal methyl methacrylate splint. *Orthop Rev* 1978; 7:25–32.

Bunch W: Muscular dystrophy, in Hardy JH (ed): *Spinal Deformity in Neurological and Muscular Disorders*. St Louis, CV Mosby Co, 1973.

Cady RB, Bobechko WP: Incidence, natural history, and treatment of scoliosis in Friedreich's ataxia. *J Pediatr Orthop* 1984; 4:673–676.

Drennan JC: Surgical management of neuromuscular scoliosis, in *Neuromuscular Diseases*. New York, Raven Press, 1984, pp 551–556.

Edelstein G: Correlation of handedness and degree of joint contracture in bilateral muscle and joint disease. *Am J Phys Med* 1959; 38:45–47.

Fowler WM: Rehabilitation management of musuclar dystrophy and related disorders: II. Comprehensive care. *Arch Phys Med Rehabil* 1982; 63:322–328.

Galasko CSB: The difficult spine. *Isr J Med Sci* 1977; 13:197–202.

Gibson DA, Wilkins KE: The management of spinal deformities in Duchenne muscular dystrophy: A new concept of spinal bracing. *Clin Orthop* 1975; 108:41–51.

Gibson DA, Albisser AM, Koreska J: Role of the wheelchair in the management of the muscular dystrophy patient. *Can Med Assoc J* 1975; 113:964–966.

Gibson DA, Koreska J, Robertson D, et al.: The management of spinal deformity in Duchenne's muscular dystrophy. *Orthop Clin North Am* 1978; 9: 437–450.

Hardy JH (ed): *Spinal Deformity in Neurological and Muscular Disorders,* ed 1. St Louis, CV Mosby Co, 1973.

Hensinger RN, MacEwen GD: Spinal deformity associated with heritable neurological conditions: Spinal muscular atrophy, Friedreich's ataxia, familial dysautonomia, and Charcot-Marie-Tooth disease. *J Bone Joint Surg* 1976; 58A:13–24.

Hsu JD: The natural history of spine curvature progression in the nonambulatory Duchenne muscular dystrophy patient. *Spine* 1983; 6:771–775.

Johnson EW, Yarnell SK: Hand dominance and scoliosis in Duchenne muscular dystrophy. *Arch Phys Med Rehabil* 1976; 57:462–464.

Kenrick MM: Certain aspects of managing patients with muscular dystrophy. *South Med J* 1965; 58: 996–999.

Knight G: Paraspinal acrylic inlays in the treatment of cervical and lumbar spondylosis and other conditions. *Lancet* 1959; 2:147–149.

Labelle H, Tohme S, Duhaime M, et al: Natural history of scoliosis in Friedrich's ataxia. *J Bone Joint Surg* 1986; 68A:504–572.

Luque E: Segmental spinal instrumentation for correction of scoliosis and paralytic scoliosis in growing children. *Clin Orthop* 1982; 163:192–204.

Luque E: *Segmental Spinal Instrumentation*. Thorofare, New Jersey, Slack, Inc, 1984.

McKenzie MW, Rogers JE: Use of trunk supports for severely paralyzed people. *Am J Occup Ther* 1973; 27:147.

Moseley CF: Natural history and management of scoliosis in Duchenne muscular dystrophy, in *Neuromuscular Diseases*. New York, Raven Press, 1984, pp 545–550.

Pecak F, Trontelj JV, Dimitrijevic MR: Scoliosis in neuromuscular disorders. *Int Orthop* 1980; 3:323–328.

Renshaw TS: Spinal fusion with segmental instrumentation. *Contemp Orthop* 1982; 4:413–419.

Rideau Y: Le traitement des dystrophies musculaires progressives: Espoir ou realite? *Quest-Medical* 1975; 28:1777–1786.

Rideau Y, Glorion B, Delanbier A, et al.: The treatment of scoliosis in Duchenne muscular dystrophy. *Muscle Nerve* 1984; 7:281–286.

Robin GC: Neurological disease and scoliosis. *Isr J Med Sci* 1973; 9:739–744.

Robin GC: Scoliosis in childhood muscular dystrophy. *J Bone Joint Surg* 1971; 53A:466–476.

Robin GC, Stein H, Simkin A, et al: The effect of methacrylate cement on loading of Harrington instruments in the spine: A preliminary experimental study. *Med Biol Eng* 1974; 12:241–245.

Sakai DN, Hsu JD, Bonnett CA, et al: Stabilization of the collapsing spine in Duchenne muscular dystrophy. *Clin Orthop* 1977; 128:256–260.

Schwentker EP, Gibson DA: The orthopaedic aspects of spinal muscular atrophy. *J Bone Joint Surg* 1976; 58A: 32–38.

Seeger BR, Sutherland A, Clark MS: Orthotic management of scoliosis in Duchenne muscular dystrophy. *Arch Phys Med Rehabil* 1984; 65:83–86.

Shapiro F, Bresnan M: Current concepts review: Orthopaedic management of childhood neuromuscular disease. *J Bone and Joint Surg* 1982; 64A:1102–1107.

Siegel IM: Scoliosis in muscular dystrophy. *Clin Orthop* 1973; 93:235–238.

Siegel IM: Problem of scoliosis management in neuromuscular disease, in Serratrice G (ed): *Neuromuscular Diseases*. New York, Raven Press, 1984, pp 535–537.

Wilkins KE, Gibson DA: The patterns of spinal deformity in Duchenne muscular dystrophy. *J Bone Joint Surg* 1976; 58:24–32.

20

Fractures

"Treat the patient, not the x-ray."
James M. Hunter (1924–), Address, American Fracture Association,
October, 1964.

It is said that muscular dystrophy is a disease where the soft tissues get hard and the hard tissues get soft. Fractures in patients with myopathy are incurred secondary to bone atrophy caused by lack of muscle tension related to decrease in muscle volume, as well as disuse osteoporosis. No aberrations of bone mineral metabolism have been found. The incidence of fracture increases with the severity of the disease, and the most severe fractures are seen in wheelchair patients who fall from the chair rather than in patients still ambulatory.

I. The metaphyses of long bones are most frequently broken, the humerus and femur most commonly involved.
II. There is usually minimal displacement of bone fragments and often less pain than with a fracture in a normal child because there is little muscle spasm.
III. Such fractures should heal without complication within the expected time interval.
IV. The danger of restrictive procedures in children with DMD must be recognized and their fractures *treated with minimal splintage.*

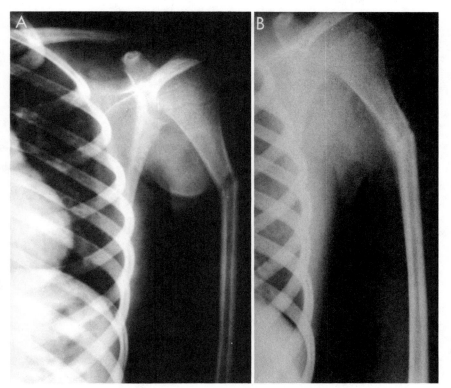

FIG 20–1.
A, fracture of humeral shaft. **B,** healing after three weeks of treatment with light plaster mold and sling.

A. Light long leg walking cast for femoral fracture, light plaster mold and sling for humeral fracture, etc. (Figs 20–1 to 20–4).
B. Femoral neck fractures should be treated by internal fixation followed by pool ambulation to avoid disuse atrophy. Because of weak shoulder girdle stabilizers, crutches are not useful.
C. The key to success is "less is more," use light support—maintain ambulation.

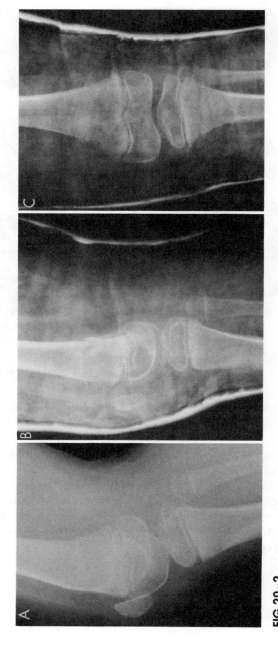

FIG 20–2.
A, fracture of distal femur. **B** and **C,** reduction and immobilization in light walking plaster.

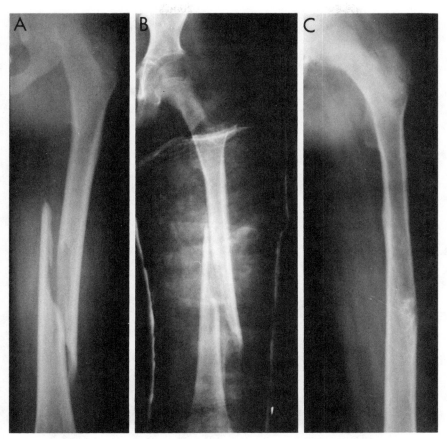

FIG 20–3.
A, fracture of femoral shaft. **B,** no attempt at reduction-walking plaster. **C,** healing and remodeling after one year.

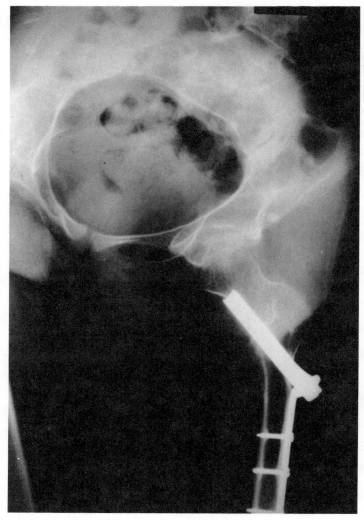

FIG 20–4.
Open reduction-internal fixation for subtrochanteric fracture, followed by prolonged bed rest. The fracture healed, but the patient never walked again. Note metal cutting out the inferior femoral neck.

BIBLIOGRAPHY

Hirotani H, et al.: Fractures in patients with myopathies. *Arch Phys Med Rehabil* 1979; 60:178–182.
Hsu JD, Garcia-Ariz M: Fracture of the femur in the Duchenne muscular dystrophy patient. *J Pediatr Orthop* 1981; 1:203–207.
Siegel IM: Fractures of long bones in Duchenne muscular dystrophy. *J Trauma* 1977; 17:219–222.
Spencer GE, Jr: Orthopedic considerations in the management of muscular dystrophy, in Ahstrom JP (ed): *Current Practice in Orthopedic Surgery*, vol 5. St Louis, CV Mosby Co, 1978.

21

Occupational Therapy

"To cure sometimes, to relieve often, to comfort always."

Anonymous

The occupational therapist can aid in assessing and assisting the patient with muscular dystrophy who finds it increasingly difficult to attend to his tasks of daily living. This assessment is directed toward testing to determine the level of self-care independence (Fig 21–1). In this regard, upper extremity range of motion and muscle strength are of special importance. Teaching gross and fine motor coordination exercises for self-care training as well as providing adaptive equipment as needed fall within the purview of occupational therapy. An evaluation of the home environment can provide the therapist with useful information concerning the patient's practical needs, and proper follow-up helps insure compliance in the use of prescribed equipment.

I. The diagnostic period. At the time of diagnosis (usually 3–4 years of age), problems of parental overprotectiveness must be considered. Developmental testing and evaluation of play behavior are important. The OT program at this stage mostly involves family education with supervision of age-appropriate activities.

II. Early childhood (5–7 years of age). The major problems here are:
A. Inability to keep up with peers during play.

OCCUPATIONAL THERAPY ASSESSMENT

Name: _____

Age: _____

Diagnosis: _____

Hand Dominance: _____

	Right					Left		
Type of Prehension:	DATE	DATE	DATE	DATE	DATE	DATE	DATE	DATE
Gross Grasp								
Translation								
Lateral Pinch								
Tip Pinch								
3 Jaw Chuck								
Prehension with:	DATE	DATE	DATE	DATE	DATE	DATE	DATE	DATE
Wrist Extended								
Wrist Flexed								

Name: _____

Address: _____ Date:_____

Name: _____

Address: _____ Date:_____

Name: _____

Address: _____ Date:_____

Name: _____

Address: _____ Date:_____

Date: _____ Birthdate: _____

Diagnosis: _____ Appliance: _____

Therapist: _____

Code: G: Able to perform activity independently

Y: Able to perform with one assist, adaptive device, partial performance, too much time

R: Cannot do

NA: Not applicable

NT: Not tested

FIG 21–1.

Occupational therapy assessment.   *continued.*

CLASSIFICATION	AGE*	INVENTORY LIST	DATE	REMARKS	DATE	REMARKS	DATE	REMARKS
Wheelchair	4	Forward 20 feet						
	4	Backward 5 feet						
	5	Lock, unlock brakes						
	5	Ft. rests and flaps						
Transfers	3	To bed						
	3	From bed						
	3	To chair (st. or arm)						
	3	From chair						
	4	To toilet						
	4	From toilet						
	6	To tub						
	6	From tub						
	3½	Manipulate clothing (Toil)						
	3	Wipe self						
Personal Hygiene	3½	Wash upper extremities						
	3½	Wash lower extremities						
	4	Brush teeth						
	5	Comb hair						
		Shave/Makeup						
	4	Open jars, tubes, etc.						
	3	Turn faucets on and off						
Dressing	3	Shoes						
	2	Shoes off						
	5	Tie shoes						
	2½	Socks on						
	2	Socks off						
	3	Unbutton shirt						
	4½	Button shirt						
	4	Put shirt on						
	2½	Take shirt off						
	4	Pullover on						
	2½	Pullover off						
	3	Pants on						
	2	Pants off						
	4	Fasten pants						
	3	Unfasten pants						
	4½	Buckle belt						
	3½	Hat on and off						
	2½	Mittens/Gloves						
	4½	Coat on and off						
		Brace, prosthesis, splint						

*Age at which task is normally performed.

FIG 21–1 *(cont.)*

CLASSIFICATION	AGE*	INVENTORY LIST	DATE	REMARKS	DATE	REMARKS	DATE	REMARKS
Feeding	2	Drink from cup (full)						
	3	Drink from glass (full)						
	2½	Drink from straw						
	3	Utensil feed						
	6	Cut with a knife						
		Special feeding device						
Miscellaneous		Glasses on and off						
		Pick up items from floor						
		Telephone						
		Write name and address						

History: _____

_____

_____

Schooling: _____

Avocation and Sports Interests: _____

Adaptive Equipment: _____

_____

Handedness: _____

Name and Address: _____

_____

_____

Additional Comments: _____

FIG 21–1 *(concluded)*

B. Early difficulties with self-care.
C. Misunderstanding of the disease because of lack of community education. Assaying upper extremity strength is important. Intervention includes assisting the child with key problems in play, self-care, and school; establishing and maintaining school liaison to educate the community concerning the child's disease and the physical problems it imposes; structuring activities for gross motor, adaptive, and sedentary play to maximize residual strength.
III. Childhood (7–12 years of age). Still ambulatory with or without braces. This period is particularly difficult as the aims are:
A. To keep the child "mainstreamed," both in school and the community.
B. To encourage independence at home. A home visit is useful at this time to assess the living environment and determine the need for self-help aids, lifts, ramps, or other architectural modifications in the home.

C. To promote selective self-care independence both at and away from home. This may require altering expectations, particularly concerning time factors, and the use of a manual wheelchair for long distance travel. Problems of dressing and toileting are usually addressed during this stage. Functional status must be reassessed because of a decrease in gross motor skills. The patient should be instructed in the independent use of orthoses if feasible.

TABLE 21–1.
Adaptive Aids and Assistive Devices

1. Easy-lift chair	Assists patient to standing position
2. Bathroom grab bars	For standing and transfer
3. Clothing adaptations	Utilizing easily manipulated Velcro fastenings, special zippers on trousers, large socks with elastic tops, oversized-buttoned shirt, etc. for easy manipulation and facilitation of independence and self-care
4. Foot boards	To diminish heel cord contracture
5. Over-bed cradles	To keep covers off the legs for comfort, enabling the patient to move freely in bed without fighting the weight of blankets
6. Reachers	For patients with proximal weakness
7. Hydraulic or electric lifts	For use in transfer to and from chair, bed, bath, etc.
8. Inlay-depth shoes with deerskin uppers	For foot comfort and stability
9. Balanced forearm orthosis (ball-bearing feeders)	To assist feeding and other fine motor skills in wheelchair-confined patient
10. Button hooks	Of value to patient with weakness and loss of fine finger movement
11. Wrist extension splint	For wrist stability to free fingers
12. Extension-handle utensils	To eliminate need for lifting the forearm in patient with proximal weakness
13. Wheelchair cushion	Most frequently used are "eggcrate" foam, silicone gel, and solid seat foam insert
14. Alternating pressure mattress, waterbed, special foam mattress	To assist in alleviating body pressure during sleep
15. Nylon sheets and pajamas	Facilitates position changes in bed by decreasing friction of movement
16. Raised chairs or toilet seat	Requires less hip and knee extensor strength in rising
17. Doorknob extensions	Increases lever arm
18. Built-up-handle eating utensils	To provide improved grasp
19. Wheelchair lap trays	To provide conveniently placed work surface
20. Transfer boards	For sliding transfer from wheelchair to car or bed

IV. Late childhood—nonambulatory. This stage is marked by a decrease in upper extremity strength that requires increasing assistance with TDL. Overall functional assessment is important. Particular attention is paid to range of motion exercises for the arms to aid use of the upper extremities away from the body in balanced forearm orthoses. Additionally, stretching exercises for the lower extremities are encouraged, as well as a full program of respiratory care. Assistive devices, such as reachers, feeding aids, adaptive clothing, lap boards, etc., are prescribed in increasing numbers during this stage (Table 21–1 and Fig 21–2).

V. Young adulthood. This period is characterized by decreased strength and range of motion accompanied by increased contractures. Various social problems, including peer interaction, require consideration at this time. Realistic preparation for college and anticipated vocation are important. In addition to maintaining range of motion, equipment needs, including telephone aids that maintain social contact, and special adaptive equipment to com-

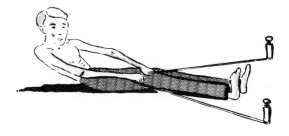

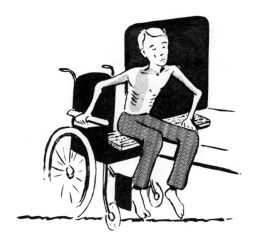

FIG 21–2.
Simple TDL aids. *Top,* rope attached to bedposts for assistance in sitting up. *Bottom,* waxed board for transfer.

pensate for severe motor loss are important. Work simplification techniques are taught. Providing a hip level "bar stool" with a back, arm rests, and foot rung makes it easier for the patient to sit and get up with minimal assistance so he will be less hesitant to socialize at home.

NOTE: The sensitive, intelligent program of occupational therapy anticipates when changes of function may occur, altering patient expectations, and programming accordingly. One must monitor the progression of the disease and functional changes, focusing on key problems as related to TDL, and staging appropriate intervention. For this, continuing familial support is required, and for that, rapport and trust are essential.

BIBLIOGRAPHY

Around-the-clock aids for the child with muscular dystrophy. Muscular Dystrophy Association of America, Inc, Pub No 146, 1977.

Cherry DB: Transfer techniques for children with muscular dystrophy. *Phys Ther* 1973; 53:970–971.

Chyatte SB, Long C, II, Vignos PJ, Jr: The balanced forearm orthosis in muscular dystrophy. *Arch Phys Med Rehabil* 1965; 46:633–636.

McKenzie MW, Rogers JE: Use of trunk supports for severely paralyzed people. *Am J Occup Ther* 1973; 27:147–148.

Morris AG, Vignos PJ, Jr: A self-care program for the child with progressive muscular dystrophy. *Am J Occup Ther* 1960; 4:301–305.

22

Nutrition

"Tell me what you eat, and I will tell you what you are."
Brillant Savarin (1755–1826)
La physiologie du gout. *Fundamental Truths* (Translated by R. E. Anderson in *Gastronomy as Fine Art*)

Dietary management is important throughout the course of muscular dystrophy. Myopathy in McArdle's syndrome, acid-maltase deficiency, and debrancher enzyme deficiency have been improved with high-protein nutrition. Kearns-Sayre syndrome has been treated with coenzyme Q10. Obesity prevention is vital in borderline neuromuscular disease patients where a slight increase in weight can seriously jeopardize ambulation. In this instance particularly, weight must be monitored at each medical contact. Individualized high quality nutrition should be provided while meeting the physical and therapeutic requisites of the disease. A well-balanced diet will provide at least 2,400 calories in an active child and 1,200 in one who is wheelchair confined. It must include adequate protein, carbohydrate, fat, vitamins, minerals, trace elements, water, and bulk.

Major problems in meeting this requirement include:

I. Inadequate growth and nutrition standards. Growth and development can be monitored (by comparing weight/height/age with standard nutritional charts) and nutritional status assessed through a nutrition history and food intake records. A normal male shows his greatest weight increment between 12–16 years in contrast with a dystrophic male whose greatest increment occurs between 10–13 years, after which his weight will usually level or decrease. Nutrition education should be provided to parents and/ or patients (e.g., the four basic food groups: (Fig 22–1) milk, meat, fruit/vegetable, grain; avoiding too much fat, saturated fat, cholesterol, sugar, salt). Adequate vitamin and mineral (particularly calcium) consumption should be stressed (this may require supplementation). Fiber and fluid intake are emphasized. Serial dietary evaluations and clinical and biochemical profiles can point out early nutritional deficiency states.

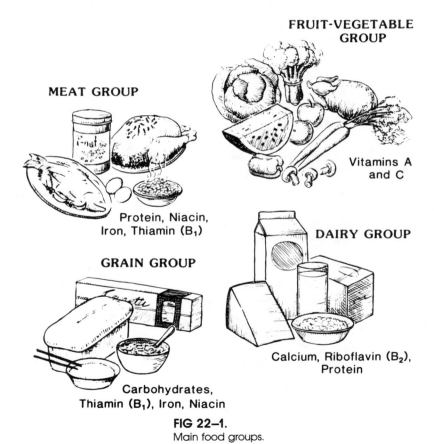

FRUIT-VEGETABLE
GROUP

MEAT GROUP

Vitamins A
and C

Protein, Niacin,
Iron, Thiamin (B$_1$)

DAIRY GROUP

GRAIN GROUP

Calcium, Riboflavin (B$_2$),
Protein

Carbohydrates,
Thiamin (B$_1$), Iron, Niacin

FIG 22–1.
Main food groups.

II. Physiological or mechanical causes for feeding disability (Fig 22–2).
  A. Feeding technique.
    1. Decreased ability to suck.
      a) Treat by spooning food.
    2. Decreased proprioception or weak grasp leading to inability to bring food to mouth.
      a) Treat through the use of long eating implements, BFAO, and other feeding aids.
    3. Improperly prepared food.
      a) Treat by providing softened, pureed or liquid foods.
  B. Difficulty with swallowing is seen in ALS patients with bulbar signs. Patients in the later stages of muscular dystrophy find deglutition difficult because of posterior pharyngeal and up-

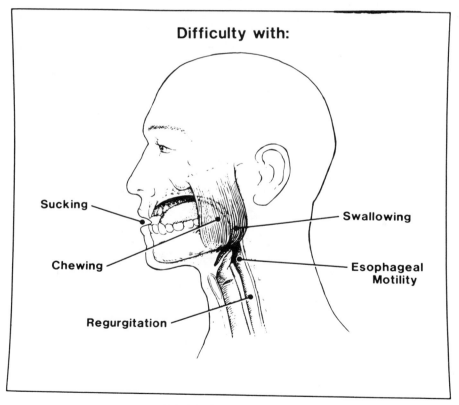

Difficulty with:

Sucking

Chewing

Regurgitation

Swallowing

Esophageal Motility

FIG 22–2.
Causes of feeding disability.

per esophageal weakness. Oculopharyngeal myopathy (a rare autosomal dominant muscle disease) is characterized by dysphagia. Patients with myotonic dystrophy or paramyotonia should avoid cold foods or fluids because they may provoke pharyngeal myotonia.

1. Chewing weakness.
    a) Treat with foods requiring less vigorous chewing.
2. Palatal weakness.
    a) Thicker liquids are easier to swallow than thin ones. A patient with palatal weakness may swallow a malted milk easier than a glass of water.
3. Decreased esophageal motility(Fig 22–3). The upper third of the esophagus is striated muscle, the middle third mixed, and only the lower third entirely smooth muscle. Problems of deglutition may result because of involvement of both voluntary and involuntary musculature. Dysfunc-

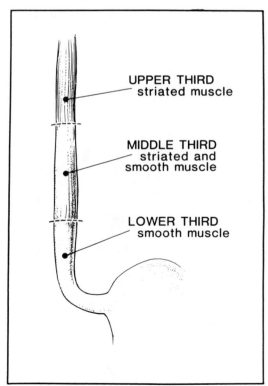

FIG 22–3.
Esophageal anatomy.

UPPER THIRD
striated muscle

MIDDLE THIRD
striated and
smooth muscle

LOWER THIRD
smooth muscle

tion of smooth muscle, particularly that of the GI tract, has been found in muscular dystrophy. Both acute megacolon and gastric dilatation have been reported. Treatment of these conditions is no different than in the patient without muscle disease. The following gastrointestinal problems have been reported in DMD (apparently secondary to smooth muscle involvement):

  a) Pharynx.
    (1) Weak or absent cricopharyngeal sphincter.
    (2) Positive vallecular sign.
    (3) Aspiration.
  b) Esophagus.
    (1) Decreased, uncoordinated, or nonperistaltic stripping.
    (2) Dilated esophagus.
    (3) Delay at the esophagogastric junction.
  c) Stomach.
    (1) Distention.
    (2) Atony.
    (3) Altered peristalsis.
  d) Small bowel.
    (1) Obstruction.
    (2) Malabsorption.
    (3) Ileus.
  e) Colon.
    (1) Dilatation.
    (2) Pseudo-obstruction.
    (3) Volvulus.
  f) Gallbladder.
    (1) Decreased contractility.
    (2) Increased incidence of cholelithiasis.
C. Regurgitation.
  1. Gastroesophageal reflux may occur.
    a) Treat with instruction in eating slowly, introducing soft and pureed foods into the diet, sitting upright for a time after meals, avoiding excessive fluids with meals, not eating a heavy meal close to bedtime, sleeping in a propped-up position. Atropine-like drugs can also be used.
  2. Aspiration.
    a) Instruction in proper positioning (head and neck flexion) to assist gravity by straightening the esophagus.

Tube feedings, esophagostomy, gastrostomy, and suction when indicated because of weakness (Table 22–1).

D. Gastric distention due to excessive solute in meal, severe bulbar symptoms in ALS, or too much atropine-like medications.

    1. Treat by removing inciting factor where feasible.

III. Obesity occurs particularly after wheelchair confinement and hastens functional disability. Many children handle their anxiety by excessive eating. Well-meaning but ignorant caretakers handle theirs by excessive feeding. It is easier to prevent this complication than to treat it.

A. The obese patient should be provided a well-balanced vitamin-supplemented diet of no less than 1,200 calories. Patients are encouraged to choose fruits and vegetables as an alternative to high-calorie snacks. High-fiber foods and fruit juices aid in maintaining normal elimination. Only small amounts of milk products are offered because of their mucus-producing tendency.

    1. Wheelchair-bound patients often reduce fluid intake and, reluctant to ask for toileting assistance, retain urine as long as possible. Such urinary stasis predisposes to infection. In addition to assuring adequate fluid intake, foods such as cereals, meats, poultry, fish, and cranberry juice, which lower urinary pH because of their acid residues, are advised.

B. Where undernutrition is a problem, daily food intake can be

---

TABLE 22–1.
Swallowing Instructions*

Positioning: Essential. Sit upright (in chair, if possible) with hips flexed at 90-degree angle (this is the best mechanical posture to route food over trachea into the esophagus). Head and trunk should be in midline position.

Flexion of head when swallowing: actively or passively bend chin slightly toward chest when swallowing.

Allow enough time to eat. Feed or take small bites of food and sips of liquid.

Conversation may be distracting when eating. Be cautious and aware of when you talk.

Watch or listen for a swallow after each mouthful or spoonful has entered.

"Flushing" some foods with liquid can cause aspiration if it is not done carefully.

Don't eat when lethargic or tired.

Look for any remains of food in mouth after eating.

Remain sitting for 10–15 minutes after eating.

---

*Routine: Place food in mouth, hold, close lips, tilt chin toward chest, swallow. If you feel as though you swallowed wrong, immediately cough, then swallow again. If routine doesn't work, chew on a few teaspoons of ice chips before eating.

supplemented with dietary additives containing low-
potassium hyperalimentatic middle-chain triglycerides.
IV. Constipation. Due to inactivity, problem with GI transit time or
other gastrointestinal dysfunction, decreased fluid and fiber intake (use of low-fiber, highly refined foods), poor meal pattern-

TABLE 22–2.
Potassium*

Foods	Potassium (mg)
½ avocado	605
Prune juice†	430
5–6 dried peach halves with juice	430
½ of 4½" cantaloupe or muskmelon	375
1 small banana	370
Orange juice, canned or fresh†	365
6 medium prunes	350
Orange juice‡	345
Grapefruit and orange juice†	335
Tangerine juice†	325
Grapefruit and orange juice‡	320
Tangerine juice‡	315
Grapefruit juice‡	310
Blackberry juice†	310
2 medium Damson plums	300
½ slice watermelon, 6" diam. and 1½" thick	300
Grapefruit juice, canned or fresh†	295
2 medium nectarines	295
Apricot nectar†	275
Tomato juice, low sodium†	270
Pineapple juice†	270
Pineapple juice‡	250
1 small tomato	245
4 canned apricot halves and 2 tbsp. juice	240
5–6 medium kumquats	235
1 oz. package of raisins	230
Grape juice†	210
⅓ cup cooked rhubarb	205
⅔ black raspberries	200
1 small orange	200
1 medium peach	200
Apple juice†	185

*Values in or calculated (rounded to the nearest 5) from Composition
of Foods—Raw, Processed, Prepared. *United States Department of Ag-
riculture Handbook,* No. 8, Revised, December, 1963.
†6 oz. canned juice.
‡Concentrated juice diluted as directed, 6 oz.
Foods with liberal amounts of potassium are required by some people,
due to certain medical treatments. The above sources (listed in order of
their value) have the largest amount of potassium and are the easiest
to add to the diet. These foods are also low in sodium.

TABLE 22–3.
The Two- to Three-Gram
Sodium Diet

This diet is a full diet with the omission of the salt shaker at table and highly salted foods. A small amount of salt may be used in cooking. The foods listed are eliminated.

Potato chips	Meat stock soups
Mustard	Gravies
Pickles	Pork
Salted nuts	Pork products
Olives	Luncheon meats
Catsup	Salted crackers

ing, poor toileting habits, and hypokalemia (fecal impaction is a complication of terminal muscle disease). Treat with:

A. Whole grain cereals.
B. Fresh vegetables (pureed) and foods high in methylcellulose.
C. Increased fluid intake.
D. Natural laxatives (prunes, stewed fruits, etc.).
E. Increased activity, regulation of meal pattern, and encouraging patient to respond to evacuation urge.
F. Diarrhea may be due to impaction, solute overload, lactase deficiency, laxative abuse, or certain antacids. Treat by removing the causative stimulus and providing antidiarrheic.
G. Rectal prolapse can occur secondary to anal sphincter weakness.
H. Drug-related malnutrition. Many medications alter absorption and/or metabolism of nutrients and minerals. Examples follow:

Drug	Purpose	Nutrients Affected
Mineral oil	Laxative	Vitamins A, D, K
Phenobarbital Dilantin	Anticonvulsants	Calcium
Antacids	Antiacidic	Phosphates
Aminophylline	Muscle relaxant, respiratory stimulant and diuretic	Sodium

Tables 22–2 and 22–3, respectively, list foods containing liberal amounts of potassium and a simplified 2–3-gm sodium diet. This information is valuable in the management of patients on steroids.

BIBLIOGRAPHY

Clydesdale F, Francis F: *Food, Nutrition, and You.* Englewood Cliffs, New Jersey, Prentice-Hall, Inc, 1977.

Consumer's Guide (eds): *The Vitamin Book.* New York, Simon and Schuster, Inc, 1979.

Gilbert S: *You Are What You Eat.* New York, Macmillan Publishing Co, 1977.

Guthrie H: *Introductory Nutrition,* ed 4. St. Louis, CV Mosby Co, 1979.

Lowenberg M, Todhunter E, Wilson E, et al: *Food and People,* ed 3. New York, John Wiley & Sons, 1979.

Mulder D: (ed): *The Diagnosis and Treatment of Amyotrophic Lateral Sclerosis.* Boston, Houghton Mifflin Co, 1980.

Ogasahara S, et al: Treatment of Kearns-Sayre syndrome with coenzyme Q10. *Neurology* 1986; 36:45–53.

Siegel IM: *The Clinical Management of Muscle Disease.* London, William Heinemann Medical Books Ltd, 1977.

Siegel IM: The management of muscular dystrophy: A clinical review. *Muscle Nerve* 1978; 1:453–460.

Slonim AE, Coleman RA, Moses WS: Myopathy and growth failure in debrancher enzyme deficiency: Improvement with high-protein nocturnal enteral therapy. *J Pediatr* 1984; 105:906–911.

Slonim AE, Goans PJ: Myopathy in McArdle's syndrome (improvement with a high-protein diet). *N Engl J Med* 1985; 312:355–359.

Slonim AE, et al: Improvement of muscle function in acid maltase deficiency by high-protein therapy. *Neurology* 1983; 33:34–38.

Slonim AE, et al: Reversal of debrancher deficiency myopathy by the use of high-protein nutrition. *Ann Neurol* 1982; 11:420–422.

23

Cardiac

"Of all the ailments which may blow out life's little candle, heart disease is the chief."

William Boyd, *Pathology for the Surgeon*

Cardiomyopathy is a complication of all forms of muscular dystrophy. It is common in DMD (50%–85% of patients eventually show clinical cardiac involvement); it may be seen in limb-girdle dystrophy; it has been found (though rarely) in FSH. Though uncommon in Becker's dystrophy, certain kindreds have serious dystrophic cardiomyopathy, and these patients stand a significant risk of sudden cardiac death. It is occasionally seen in the recessive form of DMD. Ninety percent of patients with Friedreich's ataxia show cardiac abnormalities. Conduction defects are frequently found in dystrophia myotonica and also can be seen in Refsum's disease.

Heart block is part of the clinical picture of ophthalmoplegia, retinitis pigmentosa, skeletal deformity, mental retardation, and cardiac abnormalities in the Kearns-Sayre syndrome. Nonspecific ST-T wave changes, as well as varying degrees of A-V block (including bundle branch block), right and left axis deviation, and left atrial complex abnormalities can be found in polymyositis. Cardiac arrhythmias, congestive heart failure, coronary arteritis, and myocarditis have also been reported in inflammatory myopathy.

294

I. Types of cardiac dysfunction exhibited in neuromuscular disease:
  A. Myocardial failure.
  B. Mitral valve prolapse.
  C. Conduction disturbances.
II. Cardiomyopathy in Duchenne muscular dystrophy.
  A. Although most patients with DMD die of inanition and pulmonary infection, cardiomyopathy is an important contributory cause of death. Such disease may be simulated, aggravated, or obscured by weakness of the chest bellows and diaphragm, or deformity of the thorax and recurrent lower respiratory infection. Dyspnea, fatigue, and tachycardia are provoked by muscular effort. Sudden episodes of palpitation, diaphoresis, abdominal pain, or emesis may occur. However, the patient may not show clinical evidence of heart disease (even though cardiomyopathy is noted on the electrocardiogram), restricted activity maintaining a precarious clinical status quo. Rapidly progressive preterminal heart failure often occurs after years of such clinical stability. Thoracic deformity and an elevated diaphragm make physical and x-ray examination of the heart difficult.

   Both myocardial systolic and diastolic dysfunction are noted. Symptoms of congestive failure may be masked by the severity of skeletal muscle involvement. Patients with advanced myopathy, particularly when wheelchair confined, often compensate for severe lumbar lordosis by flattening their normal thoracic kyphosis. A "straight back syndrome" can occur that may mimic organic heart disease by causing a systolic murmur due to impingement on or distortion of the great vessels and cardiac compression secondary to decrease in anteroposterior chest diameter. This may result in pseudocardiomegaly and/or an abnormal electrocardiogram. Recognition of this "pseudo heart disease" can avoid overtreatment.
  B. Auscultatory findings in DMD may include:
    1. Basal ejection murmur.
    2. Increased incidence of third and fourth sounds (quadruple rhythm).
    3. Occasionally the murmur of mitral regurgitation secondary to dystrophic involvement of a papillary muscle or adjacent myocardium (mitral valve prolapse in DMD is an expression of underlying cardiomyopathy of the papillary muscles and is age-related). This may disappear with treatment and can be confused with the murmur of tricus-

pid regurgitation in patients with right heart involvement or strain.

4. S3 and/or S4: The incidence increases with the duration of the disease.
5. Wide split S2.
6. Kyphoscoliosis may influence physical findings and a midsystolic click (which is found with mitral valve prolapse) can be associated with this skeletal deformity.
7. Late systolic murmur (uncommon).
8. Late congestive failure.
9. Dysrhythmias* (EKG-confirmed).
    a) Labile sinus tachycardia.
    b) Premature beats (atrial or ventricular).
    c) Atrial flutter.
    d) Paroxysmal ventricular tachycardia.
    e) Sinus arrhythmia.
    f) Sinus pauses.
    g) Atrial ectopic rhythm.
    h) Junctional rhythm.
10. Conduction disorders (EKG-confirmed).
    a) Abnormal intra- or interatrial conduction.
    b) Mobitz type I block.
    c) Nonconducted atrial premature beats.
    d) Short PR interval.
    e) Right ventricular conduction delay.
    f) Rightward axis compatible with left posterior fascicular block.
C. Enzyme quantification.
   1. CPK isozymes have been useful in detecting heart muscle involvement in DMD (MB fraction increased).
   2. Lactic dehydrogenase isozyme profile of dystrophic skeletal muscle resembles that of cardiac muscle, and a meaningful distinction cannot be made.
D. EKG changes. There are EKG abnormalities in up to 85% of patients, but there is little clinical correlation between the EKG and clinical status.
   1. Electrocardiograms distinctive of DMD (tall R waves in right precordial leads and deep Q waves in lateral chest leads) have sometimes been found in asymptomatic female carriers (increased R-S amplitude sums and R/S ra-

*Except for end-stage atrial flutter, the dysrhythmias and conduction disorders found in DMD are not clinically deleterious.

tios in leads V-1 and V-2 are also seen). The only other manifestation of myopathic disease noted in these carriers is an elevated CPK. Conduction abnormalities are less common and arrhythmias are rare. Vectorcardiography can sometimes detect otherwise obscure pathology in DMD. Cardiomyopathy, with or without cardiac insufficiency, may be suspected because of certain typical patterns seen on a standard 12-lead scalar EKG (Fig 23–1). These include:

a) Tall right precordial R waves with increased R/S ratios (V$_1$ and V$_3$R), which may progress to the development of incomplete right bundle branch block with eventual disappearance of the tall R wave.

b) Deep limb lead and lateral precordial Q waves (specifically seen in X-linked Duchenne dystrophy).

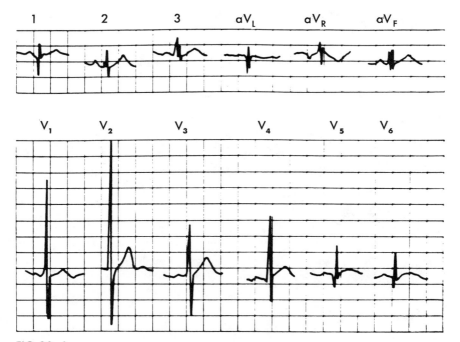

FIG 23–1.
Some typical EKG findings in cardiomyopathy (from a 14-year-old boy with Duchenne muscular dystrophy). Note: (1) narrow but deep Q waves in leads 1, aVL, V$_5$, and V$_6$; (2) RSR pattern in aVR; (3) dominant R waves in V$_1$ and V$_2$. (Modified from Walton JN (ed); *Disorders of Voluntary Muscle*, ed 3. New York, Churchill Livingstone, Inc, 1974.)

    c) Deep Q waves coexisting with an altered shape of the right precordial R wave (RSR or polyphasic R wave).

    d) At a later stage, diffuse myocardial damage may appear, manifested by inverted T waves, ST segment deviation, and abnormal Q waves.

E. Echocardiography. This technique permits investigation of the size of the cardiac chambers and the thickness of their walls. Abnormalities of systolic function are easily demonstrated, and mitral valve prolapse has been reported in 25%–50% of patients investigated by this means. Approximately one-third of patients undergoing echocardiography have shown asymmetric septal hypertrophy, hypertrophic subaortic stenosis, and left ventricular hypertrophy.

F. Myocardial pathology.

    1. The essential pathologic change (Fig 23–2) in cardiomyopathy consists of cardiac muscle atrophy, with replacement of fibers by collagenous connective tissue, blending with the sarcoplasm of adjacent cardiac muscle fibers. Fibroblastic proliferation is not present, and the cellular content

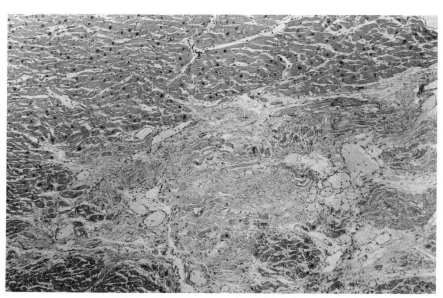

FIG 23–2.
Histopathologic changes in cardiomyopathy.

of the connective tissue probably represents surviving cardiac nuclei.

    a) Myocardial fibrosis is seen earliest and is most severe in the posterior-basal area of the left ventricle.

    b) These changes involve mostly the left ventricle, next the interventricular septum, and last the atrium. As left ventricular function decreases, global cardiac dysfunction supervenes.

    c) The conduction system can be involved, ultimately leading to sinus tachycardia and supraventricular arrhythmia.

    d) Fat replacement is not a feature of the dystrophic myocardial process.

    e) When labile sinus tachycardia occurs, it is usually due to disease of the nodal arteries. The role of the autonomic nervous system in cardiomyopathy is not entirely clear.

III. Limb-girdle dystrophy. Cardiac involvement is uncommon in this condition, but when present, it is usually expressed as:

    A. Rhythm or conduction disturbances (QRS prolongation, first-degree heart block, right ventricular conduction defects, atrial flutter).

    B. Minor T wave alterations and abnormal Q waves.

    C. Third and fourth heart sounds (quadruple rhythm).

    D. Overt cardiac failure.

IV. Cardiomyopathy and dystrophia myotonica. Findings may include:

    A. Asymptomatic EKG abnormalities.

    B. Overt rhythm and conduction disturbances.

    C. Heart failure.

    D. EKG abnormalities (which may be symptomatic).

        1. Sinus bradycardia.

        2. Slurring and prolongation of the QRS complex (left axis deviation).

        3. Left bundle branch block.

        4. Low-voltage T waves.

    E. Atrial-ventricular conduction disturbances. These are variable in this condition. Anything from mild PR interval prolongation to complete AV block has been reported. Rhythm disturbances consist chiefly of atrial flutter or fibrillation. Cardiac enlargement and sometimes heart failure may accompany DM. Systemic myotonia is clinically present long before cardiomyopathy. However, cardiac symptoms occasionally dominate the clinical picture, and cardiac involvement is sometimes responsible for sudden death. Where indicated, a demand cardiac pacemaker can be supplied. Any medication for myotonia that may affect the myocardium by slowing conduction, particularly to the distal (His bundle) system—thus increasing AV block—should be avoided. Procainamide is notorious in this regard but quinine and phenytoin (Dilantin) should also be used with caution.

   F. Ninety percent of patients with dystrophia myotonica are clinically asymptomatic for cardiomyopathy. Congestive failure occurs late. Gross examination of the heart is usually normal. The pathology consists of cardiac enlargement. Mitral valve prolapse can be found in up to 70% of patients and is unrelated to skeletal deformity.

  V. Friedreich's ataxia. Approximately 90% of patients with this condition have cardiac abnormalities. These include dysrhythmias and disorders of ventricular function as well as coronary artery disease. Most of these conditions are asymptomatic, but a patient will occasionally present with palpitation, Stokes-Adams syndrome, or even (rare) angina. Examination reveals a basal ejection murmur and the EKG shows nonspecific ST-T changes.

  VI. Management of cardiomyopathy. Disability from cardiomyopathy may be masked or may seem insignificant in comparison to that imposed by muscle weakness in neuromuscular disease. However, it may be symptomatic.

   A. Systolic function should be carefully assessed for myocardial failure. As noted above, echocardiography helps to evaluate the geometry of the heart. Vector cardiograms are also of value.

   B. For true myocardial failure, the usual management with cardiac glycosides, diuretics, and ventricular unloading in a standard manner is recommended.

   C. For diastolic dysfunction, calcium blockers such as verapamil and beta blockers such as propranolol are useful.

   D. For arrhythmias, antiarrhythmic medications as well as pacemakers are employed.

BIBLIOGRAPHY

Askari, A, Huettner T: Cardiac abnormalities in polymyositis/dermatomyositis. *Semin Arthritis Rheum* 1982; 12:208–218.

Datey KK, Deshmukh MM, Engineer SD, et al: Straight back syndrome. *Br Heart J* 1964; 26:614–619.

DeLeon AC, Jr, Perloff JK, Twigg H, et al: Straight back syndrome: Clinical cardiovascular manifestations. *Circulation* 1965; 32:193–203.

Diaz FV, Pelous AN, Valdes FG, et al: Pectus excavatum: Hemodynamic and electrocardiographic considerations (case reports). *Am J Cardiol* 1962; 10: 272–277.

Gooch AS, Maranhao V, Goldberg H, et al: The straight thoracic spine in cardiac diagnosis. *Am Heart J* 1967; 74:595–602.

Lane RJM, Gardner-Medwin D, Roses AD: Electrocardiographic abnormalities in carriers of Duchenne muscular dystrophy. *Neurology* 1980; 30:497–501.

Norris FH, Jr, Moss AJ, Yu PN: On the possibility that a type of human muscular dystrophy commences in myocardium. *Ann NY Acad Sci* 1966; 138:342–354.

Perloff JK, DeLeon AC, Jr, O'Dougherty D: The cardiomyopathy of progressive muscular dystrophy. *Circulation* 1966; 33:625–648.

Perloff JK: Cardiomyopathy associated with heredofamilial neuromyopathic diseases. *Mod Concepts Cardiovasc Dis* 1971; 40:23–26.

Perloff JK: Cardiac rhythm and conduction in Duchenne's muscular dystrophy. A prospective study of 20 patients. *J Am Coll Cardiol* 1984; 3:1263–1268.

Rawlings MS: The straight back syndrome: A new cause of pseudoheart disease. *Am J Cardiol* 1960; 5:333–338.

Reusch CS: Hemodynamic studies in pectus excavatum. *Circulation* 1961; 24:1143–1150.

Siegel IM: Cardiomyopathy: Presenting symptom of progressive muscular dystrophy. *JAMA* (letters) 1972; 222:1060.

Siegel JS, Schecter E: The straight back syndrome: Another cause of innocent systolic murmurs. *Am J Med* 1967; 42:309–313.

Slucka C: The electrocardiogram in Duchenne progressive muscular dystrophy. *Circulation* 1968; 38:933–940.

Streib EW, Meyers DG, Sun SF: Mitral valve prolapse in MyD. *Muscle Nerve* 1985; 8:650–653.

Teplick GJ, Drake EH: The roentgen and cardiac manifestations of funnel chest. *Am J Roentgenol* 1946; 56:721–735.

24

Respiratory

"A medical chest specialist is long-winded about the short-winded."
Kenneth Bird (1917–)

Pulmonary problems frequently complicate the advanced stages of neuromuscular disease. Decreased pulmonary function, compounded by poor respiratory toilet and weakness of deglutition (increasing the danger of aspiration pneumonitis), provides fertile ground for pulmonary complications, particularly hypostasic pneumonitis. Eaton-Lambert syndrome is characterized by a specific weakness pattern plus oat cell carcinoma of the lung. The malignant neoplasm seen in adult dermatomyositis is often bronchogenic carcinoma. Cardiopulmonary abnormalities encountered in dystrophia myotonia are complicated by chest wall and diaphragm myotonia and swallowing disturbances.

The diaphragm performs approximately two-thirds of the work of inspiration (ordinary expiration is a passive activity). Other force generators contributing to vital capacity are the accessory muscles of respiration. Forced expiration (also coughing and sneezing) requires abdominal as well as diaphragmatic strength to lift the diaphragm. The diaphragm weakens early in LGD, late in DMD. Diaphragmatic paralysis in ALS causes supine hypoventilation early and ultimately prevents the patient from breathing when sitting. Paradoxical abdominal respiration can be seen in ALS, also in SMA, LGD, acid-maltase deficiency, polio, and myasthenia gravis. Even a 50% VC is insufficient to support life if voluntary control is lacking. Bulbar involvement in ALS with decreased ability to cough, increased risk of aspiration, CO_2 retention, and increased metabolic load seriously compromise pulmonary function.

The three major factors influencing respiration in DMD are respiratory muscle power, thoracic growth, and degree of thoracic scoliosis. The first two peak at age 12 (when scoliosis often begins), declining thereafter, particularly with wheelchair confinement. In DMD, the first serious respiratory episode is usually atelectasis and often reversible. Maximal expiratory pressure and forced expiratory volume are the most sensitive indicators of early respiratory compromise. Examination should include a careful auscultation of the base of the lungs where crackling may indicate early atelectasis. Forced expiratory wheezing is a sign of early restrictive disease.

To breathe well, one must swallow and cough well. (Cough flow velocity may reach 500 miles per hour.) The upper respiratory tract is commonly the site of chronic upper airway obstruction. Swallowing dysfunction can lead to aspiration with subsequent pneumonitis.

Normally, 5% of available calories are used for breathing. This metabolic cost is increased with obesity and kyphoscoliosis. The muscles of respiration must work to overcome: (1) the elastic recoil of the tracheobronchial tree and the lungs; (2) alveolar surface tension; and (3) the functional resistance of the respiratory surfaces to inspired air. Respiratory problems include: (1) impaired cough; (2) atelectasis with infection; (3) hypoventilation; (4) respiratory failure—PO_2 less than 60 mm Hg and/or PCO_2 greater than 50 mm Hg.

I. Pneumonia.
   A. Secondary to inanition, decreased pulmonary function, and poor respiratory toilet with aspiration.
   B. A frequent occurrence in advanced cases of muscular dystrophy and the most common cause of death.
      1. Sudden demise in patients with dystrophic myocardial involvement may be due to acute congestive heart failure following a sudden demand, secondary to pneumonitis, on a limited cardiac reserve.
         a) This mechanism may also play a role in sudden death, which sometimes follows episodes of abdominal pain, emesis, and diarrhea, a common complication in bedridden patients leading to dehydration and electrolyte imbalance. Such a state is poorly tolerated by the dystrophic myocardium, and sudden death may result.

     C. The pneumonias typically encountered in DMD are hypostatic, involving the left lower, right lower, and right middle lobes of the lungs.

     D. Weakness of deglutition compounds infection by increasing the danger of aspiration.

     E. Debility of the oropharynx often prevents a patient from learning to breathe with his pharynx ("frog" breathing).

     F. Poor respiratory capacity and expiratory reserve volume decrease coughing effectiveness.

         1. Antihistamine decongestants should not be prescribed as they increase mucous inspissation, further irritating the respiratory passages.

     G. Aspiration pneumonitis is a common cause of death in patients with dystrophia myotonica.

         1. Decreased vital capacity, suggesting a weakened chest bellows and restrictive ventilatory defect without obstruction, can be present. Pulmonary infections are commonly suffered because of an inability of the esophagus to adequately empty, permitting nocturnal aspiration and further pulmonary embarrassment.

II. Chronic alveolar hypoventilation.

     A. This has been reported in all major forms of muscular dystrophy.

     B. Inadequate gaseous exchange across the lungs leads to hypoxemia, retention of carbon dioxide, and respiratory acidosis.

     C. Clinical symptoms are ethanol-like and include somnolence or confusion, restlessness, shortness of breath, morning headache, blurred vision, paranoia, and diplopia.

     D. There may be various degrees of organic mental disorder with coma, asterixis (as well as other movement disorders), papilledema, irregular respiration, cyanosis, and manifestations of right heart failure.

     E. Patients often complain of nightmares, and blood pressure may be increased.

     F. Secondary polycythemia has been noted.

     G. Clinical findings are associated with increased arterial carbon dioxide tension. Under these circumstances, respiratory control is modulated primarily by the action of lowered PO_2 on the carotid receptors and, as in other chronic respiratory conditions, inhaling pure oxygen may have a deleterious effect. Cyanosis is not always present with hypoxia, requiring a significant decrease in the hemoglobin level (approximately 5 gm) for its appearance. Conversely, cyanosis may be present in the absence of hypoxemia.

H. Although sedentary patients can often function on 30% vital capacity, when VC is less than 200 cc, the patient will usually stop eating.

III. Pickwickian syndrome.

A. Alveolar hypotension with a gross reduction in the maximal expiratory pressure is a common pulmonary finding in dystrophia myotonica, and pickwickian syndrome can be seen in this disease.

B. Other related findings include insomnia, headaches, nightmares, apprehension, and hyperhidrosis.

C. Intermittent positive pressure respiration, combined with weight reduction and diuretics, is the treatment of choice in these patients.

IV. Management. The major goals in respiratory care are the maintenance of pulmonary homeostasis through training in the use of various types of breathing aids, enabling the patient to lead as active and comfortable a life as possible within the limits imposed by his evolving respiratory problems. Periodic evaluation of pulmonary function to monitor restrictive pulmonary disease must be an integral part of any treatment program for patients with muscular dystrophy. Reduction of vital capacity, forced expiratory ability, and maximal voluntary ventilation are common findings. Thirty percent normal vital capacity in the chronic phase of restrictive ventilatory insufficiency can maintain tidal volume in the minimally active patient. As ventilation drops, the accessory respiratory muscles (such as the platysma and sternocleidomastoid) are brought into play. Decreased respiratory function can lead to cor pulmonale with right heart failure and cardiomyopathy. Diminished vital capacity secondary to a weakened chest bellows decreases the ability to cough. Reduction in chest compliance and progressive weakness of the pulmonary musculature require an ongoing program of pulmonary rehabilitation, including diaphragmatic breathing exercises (Table 24–1), postural drainage (Fig 24–1 and Table 24–2), proper humidification, chest percussion, and training in the use of various respiratory aids. Vigorous treatment of upper respiratory infections to avoid serious pulmonary disease should include pharyngeal suction and intermittent positive pressure breathing therapy. Mechanical ventilation of patients in the terminal stages of DMD can be managed at home with or without a tracheostomy. In the very late stages of muscu-

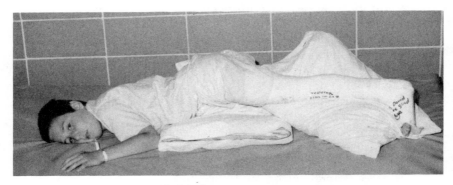

FIG 24–1.
Position for postural drainage.

lar dystrophy, there is a significant loss of ventilation with ineffective cough. At this time, minor respiratory infections can be devastating. Fear and fatigue contribute to peripheral respiratory failure. Objective signs include secondary polycythemia, elevated heart rate, increase in CO_2 combining power, reduced vital capacity, decreased cough force, reduced chest expansion, and a change in breathing pattern (labored hyperpnea). A hand resuscitator is useful at home to encourage hyperventilation and decrease cough. A portable home IPPB therapy unit is also advised. Later, a mechanical respirator may be necessary. In the extreme case, tracheostomy may be required to assist ventilation and relieve breathing fatigue. Permanent artificial ventilatory support can increase comfort and function in selected cases of neuromyopathic disease.

A. Mucokinesis. For proper consistency and flow of respiratory mucus, one must consider the following:
1. Adequate hydration.
2. Proper humidification (40%).
3. Expectorants (avoid antihistamines and other drying agents).
4. Aerosols.
5. Assisted cough.
6. IPPB.
7. Chest physical therapy and postural drainage.
8. In the extreme, bronchoscopy to remove mucous plugs.

B. Bronchopulmonary infection.
1. Prophylactic treatment as soon as the patient becomes wheelchair confined or otherwise restrained.

TABLE 24–1.
Technique of Diaphragmatic Breathing Given to Children*

1. Lie on the floor on your back. Now bend your knees, keeping your feet flat on the floor. Hold your hands over your abdomen. Now breathe in through your nose. Your abdomen should go out like a balloon. Try to relax your upper chest and shoulders. Do this ten times slowly.

2. Breathe again like above, only this time blow the air out through your pursed lips. Close your lips as though you were trying to whistle. Pulling the air in through your nose, your abdomen goes up. Blowing the air out through your lips, your abdomen goes down.

3. Count to yourself as you practice this way of breathing. Count to two as you breathe in through your nose. Count to four slowly as you blow out through your pursed lips. Blowing out is the most important. Use your hands on your abdomen to help press all the air out. Do this ten times slowly.

4. Put a book on your abdomen. See if you can make the book rise up as you take in air and make your abdomen round. Your abdomen should get flat again as you blow all the air out. While you are doing this, try to relax your chest and shoulders.

5. Sit up straight in a chair. Put a candle in front of you on a table, with the flame at the level of your mouth. Now hold your hands against your abdomen. Breathe in some air and let your abdomen push out against your hands. Now, blow out gently towards the flame through your pursed lips. See if you can bend the flame. As you blow, press gently on your abdomen. Move the candle away a little bit each day until it is two feet away. Can you still bend the flame?

6. Sit in a chair and put a ping-pong ball in front of you on a table. Blow out gently through your pursed lips towards the ball. Mark how far it goes. See if you can blow it a little farther the next time.

---

*To use the diaphragm effectively, the abdomen must rise with inspiration and fall with expiration. With the therapist's hands placed over the lower ribs, the patient is instructed to push the therapist's hands out with inspiration and allow them to move inward with expiration. With the patient in a supine position, the therapist places a hand or weight on the upper abdomen. Emphasis is placed on the proper sequence of diaphragmatic breathing. On inspiration, the abdomen rises first, next the lower ribs push out, finally the chest rises. All diaphragmatic breathing exercises are done with the shoulders relaxed. Patients are encouraged to relax and taught to breathe with the diaphragm, keeping the upper chest still. In the seated position, patients are instructed to sit straight with the arms abducted and on inspiration expand the chest as much as possible. On expiration the patient bends forward at the waist, bringing his arms down and across his chest, and forces a maximal expiration.

    a) Diaphragmatic breathing exercises.
    b) Deep breathing (blow bottles, incentive spirometer [Fig 24–2], balloon blowing, wind instruments).
2. Pneumovaccine should be administered.
3. A simple measurment of vital capacity can be obtained by having the patient inspire fully and count as fast as he can while expiring. The number reached before having to take

TABLE 24–2.
Chest Therapy Program*

I. Postural drainage. The body is placed in various positions to promote drainage of specific segments of the lung. When those bronchi draining a lung segment are perpendicular, gravity will assist the flow of secretions.
  A. Upper lobes, anterior segments both lungs: Semi-Fowler's position, sitting at 45-degree angle.
  B. Lingular and lateral segments, left lower lobe: Right side lying ¼ turn from supine, foot of bed elevated 12–14 inches.
  C. Posterior segments, left lower lobe: Right side lying ¼ turn from prone, foot of bed elevated.
  D. Anterior segments, both lower lobes: Supine–foot of bed elevated.
  E. Posterior segments, right lower lobe: Left side lying ¼ turn from prone, foot of bed elevated.
  F. Middle lobe, right lung: Left side lying ¼ turn from supine, foot of bed elevated.
II. Chest percussion. In this maneuver, the chest is "clapped" with cupped hands to loosen secretions adhering to broncheolar walls.
III. Chest vibration and compression. The flattened palms of the hands are placed on the chest wall. The arms and hands are vibrated while compressing the chest. This assists exhalation and encourages coughing.

*These maneuvers are helpful in mobilizing respiratory secretions. They are most effective when combined with aerosol and IPPB therapy.

another breath, multiplied by 100, gives a rough estimate of residual vital capacity.

4. Range of motion of the chest must be maintained.
5. Proper humidification is provided to avoid upper respiratory infections (particularly bronchitis), which may progress to more serious pulmonary disease.
6. Smoking is interdicted.
7. A program of postural drainage and chest therapy becomes part of the daily routine.
8. A foot-operated suction apparatus for home use may help remove secretions from the posterior pharynx.
9. A portable intermittent positive pressure breathing apparatus can prove useful (Fig 24–3).
10. Where decrease of esophageal motility is a problem, elevation of the head of the bed may prevent aspiration.
11. Adequate hydration (fluid balance) is essential.
12. Serial evaluation of pulmonary function and atelectasis.
13. Antipyretics.
14. Appropriate antimicrobials.

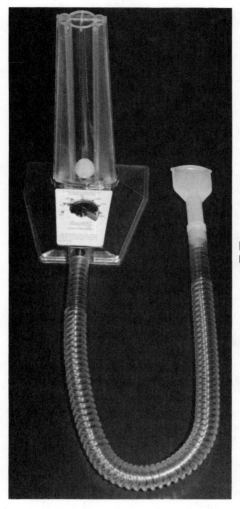

FIG 24–2.
Incentive spirometer.

   a) H influenzae and pneumococcus are the most frequent
       infecting organisms.
C. Respiratory failure. Patients in respiratory failure show dyspnea at rest or mild exertion with CO_2 retention in the absence of infection. Two types are present:
   1. Oxygen lack.
   2. CO_2 narcosis. An artificial airway with mechanical ventila-

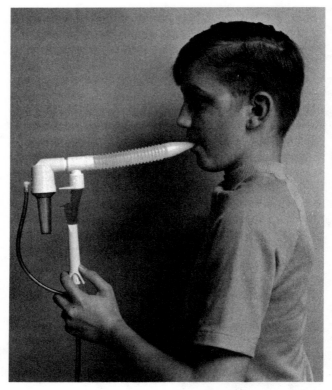

FIG 24–3.
Portable intermittent positive pressure breathing apparatus in use. (Retec NC-30, Everest and Jennings, Inc., Los Angeles).

tion to provide chronic oxygen treatment is necessary. Oxygen at home can be obtained from tanks, an electronic molecular sieve that removes nitrogen from the air, or liquid oxygen (portable). Apparatus available for late intervention mechanical ventilation includes the rocking bed, plastic wrap ventilator, pneumobelt, and chest-abdomen cuirass respirator. Positive pressure ventilators for home ventilation require a tracheostomy.

BIBLIOGRAPHY

Aberion GAA, Lee MHM, Solomon M: Pulmonary care of Duchenne type of muscular dystrophy. *NY State J Med* 1973; 73:1206–1207.

Adams MA, Chandler LS: Effects of physical therapy program on vital capacity of patients with muscular dystrophy. *Phys Ther* 1974; 54:494–496.

Adkins HV: Improvement of breathing ability in children with respiratory muscle paralysis. *Phys Ther* 1968; 48:577–581.

Alexander M, Johnson E, Petty J, et al: Mechanical ventilation of patients with late stage Duchenne muscular dystrophy: Management in the home. *Arch Phys Med Rehabil* 1979; 60:289–292.

Buschsbaum HD, Martin WA, Turino GM, et al: Chronic alveolar hypoventilation due to muscular dystrophy. *Neurology,* 1968; 18:319–327.

Burke SS, Grove NM, Houser CR, et al: Respiratory aspects of pseudo-hypertrophic muscular dystrophy. *Am J Dis Child* 1971; 121:230–234.

Dail CW: Respiratory aspects of rehabilitation in neuromuscular conditions. *Arch Phys Med Rehabil* 1965; 46:655–675.

Garrett JM, DuBose TJ, Jr, Jackson JE, et al: Esophageal and pulmonary disturbances in myotonica dystrophica. *Arch Intern Med* 1969; 123:26–32.

Greenberg M, Edmonds J: Chronic respiratory problems in neuromyopathic disorders: Their nature and management. *Pediatr Clin North Am* 1974; 21:927–934.

Houser CR, Johnson DM: Breathing exercises for children with pseudohypertrophic muscular dystrophy. *Phys Ther* 1971; 51:751–759.

Inkley SR, Oldenburg FC, Vignos PJ: Pulmonary function in Duchenne muscular dystrophy related to stage of disease. *Am J Med* 1974; 56:297–306.

McCormack WM, Spalter HD: Muscular dystrophy. Alveolar hypoventilation and papilledema. *JAMA* 1966; 197:957–960.

Neustadt JE, Levy RC, Spiegel IJ: Carbon dioxide narcosis in association with muscular dystrophy. *JAMA* 1964; 187:616–617.

Sackner MA: Diaphragmatic breathing exercises: Therapy in chronic obstructive pulmonary disease. *JAMA* 1975; 231:295–296.

Saheki B, Fukuyama K, Miyoshi M, et al: The studies on the pulmonary function of the patients of progressive muscular dystrophy. *Iryo* 1967; 21:23–30.

Siegel IM: Pulmonary problems in Duchenne muscular dystrophy: Diagnosis, prophylaxis and treatment. *Phys Ther* 1975; 55:160–162.

Vignos PJ: Respiratory function and pulmonary infection in Duchenne muscular dystrophy. *Isr J Med Sci* 1977; 13:207–214.

25

Miscellaneous Problems

"The most important thing in this hospital is me."
                            6-year-old spinal muscular atrophy patient
"This wheelchair is my home."
                            16-year-old muscular dystrophy patient

SPEECH

Dysarthrias in DMD can result from orthodontic deformity second-ary to tongue thrust (which can reach 2,000 pounds of pressure per day), changes in jaw angle (secondary to hypertrophy of masseter muscles), macroglossia, or facial muscle weakness (more than 100 mus-cles are used in speaking). Dental problems are also seen, due to mal-occlusion, weakness, and difficulty maintaining head control. Speech problems usually express themselves as (1) decreased vocal intensity, (2) reduced breath support, (3) nasality and (4) open-mouth posture. All of these may be treated through the ordinary techniques of speech therapy that can be utilized to maintain articulation skills and compen-sate for indistinctness of speech due to impaired lip, tongue, and soft palate movements (Table 25–1). Speech impairments found in specific myopathies follow.

TABLE 25–1.
Speech Therapy Exercises

I. Lip Exercises
  A. Alternate puckering and smiling, simultaneously producing oo-ee. Practice in front of a mirror.
  B. Pucker lips and fill cheeks with air. Keeping lips tightly pursed, depress inflated cheeks with fingertips and strive to keep air within the oral cavity. Do not allow any air to escape through the puckered lips, or to be swallowed.
  C. Insert a Lifesaver or button (of varying sizes) strung on dental floss between closed teeth and compressed lips. Individual should strive to retain the Lifesaver or button behind the tightly puckered lips while the therapist pulls on the dental floss, gradually increasing the resistance. This is particularly good in maintaining the strength of the orbicularis oris.
  D. Tucking the lips in until none of the red border can be seen.
  E. Puckering the lips, and moving the pursed lips from side to side as far as they will go.
  F. Compressing and releasing the lips rapidly, with the sounds *mee . . . mee . . . mee,* then changing to *pah . . . pah . . . pah, poh . . . poh . . . poh, bee . . . bee . . . bee,* and *wah . . . wah . . . wah.*
II. Tongue Exercises
  A. Mrs. Tongue Story or Circus Acts (done in front of mirror).
  B. Lingual lateralization.
III. Palatal Exercises
  A. Blowing exercises are effective in maintaining the function of the palatal muscles: Blowing bubbles in water through a straw, balloons, toy horns, whistles, a ping-pong ball or a feather across a table, and pinwheels. Also, blowing a toy boat in a pan of water or in the bathtub, using the sound oo (as in boot).
  B. Repeating syllables: *Ung-gah, ung-gah, ung-gah,* with the mouth open and no movement of the jaws.
  C. Letting the child feel the difference between nasal and mouth sounds by placing his fingers on the bridge of your nose. Sing *m-m-m-m,* then sing *ah-ah.*
  D. Emphasizing the fact that only m, n, and ng come through the nose by having the child feel the bridge of his nose as he pretends to be a humming top and says *m-m-m,* then changes to *ah . . ..*
  E. Practicing word lists for rapid adjustment from nasalized to non-nasalized sounds (i.e., sambo, ramble, amber, tamper, lamp).

I. FSH.
  A. Misarticulated sounds and substitutions due to omissions and distortions of labial sounds (P, B, M, W) owing to orbicularis oris weakness. L and T are problematic with lingual dysarthria.
  B. Sensorineural hearing loss has also been reported in FSH.
II. Advanced DMD.
  A. Diminished diodochokinetic rates of tongue and jaw movements.

B. Moderate to severe articular disorders: weakness of mandibular and lingual muscles.
C. "Dystrophic voice:" thin vocal quality with excessive nasality (weakness of velopharyngeal muscles).
D. Laryngeal impairment leading to inability to cough, clear throat, or sustain phonation.
E. Diminished vocal intensity (respiratory muscle weakness).
F. Protruded tongue and open mouth posture.
III. Oculo- or oculopharyngeal myopathy.
A. Dysphonia and dysphagia because of weakness of oropharyngeal muscles.
IV. Dystrophia myotonica (particularly the neonatal form).
A. Nasal, indistinct voice (perhaps secondary to slow myotonic relaxation of tongue muscles following strong voluntary contraction).
B. Oropharyngeal weakness can affect speech.
C. Sustained downward displacement of soft palate during speech or swallowing (myotonia of tensor veli palatini) causes nasality.
D. Sensorineural hearing loss may occur.

SKIN

Changes in the collagen vascular system of the skin have been described. Nonspecific changes in subcutaneous fat have been reported. Dermatologic pathology in DMD includes (1) a subcuticular reticular vascular pattern (livedo reticularis) accentuated by exercise, (2) erythema ab igne, and (3) seborrheic dermatitis (common).

PREGNANCY

Patients with DMD seldom procreate. On the rare occasion that this might occur, if the female is normal, all male children will be normal and all females carriers. If perchance the female in such a mating is a carrier, each child (male or female) born will be at 50% risk of inheriting the disease.

I. In the adult forms of myopathy (LGD, FSH), pregnancy is usually uneventful, though there is an occasional increased loss of muscle power during the third trimester. Because the myometrium is unaffected, labor is usually normal.

II. In dystrophia myotonica, the first stage of labor is often prolonged and assistance is often required during the second stage. Weakness and myotonia may increase. There is an increased incidence of prematurity, fetal death, spontaneous abortion, labor dysfunction, postpartum hemorrhage, hydramnios, reduced fetal movements, retained placenta, anesthetic sensitivity, and neonatal mortality.

WHEELCHAIR CARE

When ambulation is no longer possible, wheelchair confinement becomes necessary. This is a critical incident, both physiologically and psychologically, in the life of the patient with muscular dystrophy. Every effort should be devoted to making the wheelchair a passport to more, rather than less, activity. Wheelchair confinement does not signal the "beginning of the end," only "a new beginning." Special wheelchair adaptations can increase comfort while providing spinal support. Wheelchair prescription should not be regarded casually. The wheelchair is an orthosis and should be treated as such. Proper fit is vital. If it is too wide, the patient will lean to one side, facilitating the development of scoliosis; if too deep, a kyphotic posture is encouraged. Seating includes standardized modules and custom contoured seating systems (Fig 25–1).

Adequate trunk support can position the patient upright, enabling him to use a wheelchair more effectively. A firm seat and back and a wide safety belt are provided. Where weak neck extension is a prob-

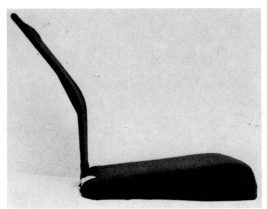

FIG 25–1.
Custom wheelchair insert to provide lordosis.

lem, an extended back rest is fitted to support the head. Further wheel-chair adaptations include (1) balanced forearm orthoses, enabling weakened upper extremity musculature to operate across rather than against the field of gravity (Fig 25–2), thus facilitating the use of the hands for self-feeding, writing, and other utilitarian tasks, and (2) lap boards to provide a comfortably positioned work surface.

The wheelchair must be of proper size with the narrowest seat width possible that gives full support. It should be the correct height from the floor. It should incorporate large roll wheels, handbrakes, adjustable, removable, elevating swinging footrests (Fig 25–3) with heel straps, located so there is no pressure behind the knees, upholstered removable desk-like arms and good brakes. The back support must not inhibit shoulder or elbow motion while it balances the trunk over the hips. A zippered back permits obese patients to be easily placed in the supine position for part of the day to stretch out hip contractures. Hamstring tightness can lead to hip extensor contracture, which in turn causes pelvic rotation and sacral sitting. Thus, the thoracolumbar spine is forced into kyphosis and the head is thrust forward. Because

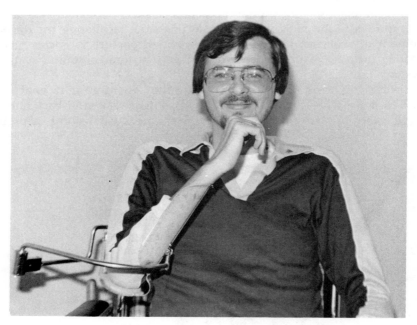

FIG 25–2.
Balanced forearm orthosis (BFAO).

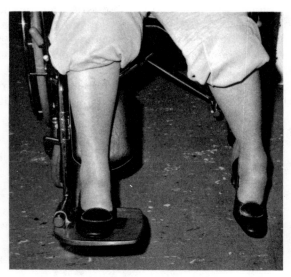

FIG 25–3.
The feet must rest on the wheelchair footrests, or Achilles contracture will occur.

of this, hamstring tightening is the major culprit in pelvic displacement for the wheelchair confined.

A combination wheelchair-commode eliminates the problem of difficult toilet transfer. Daily passive stretch of hips, knees, and ankles, augmented by foot wedges holding the ankles in neutral or dorsiflexion and extended leg rests used to prevent flexion contracture of the knees, can delay disabling contractures of the lower extremities. As long as the legs are kept supple through stretching, long leg braces can be applied and the patient easily tilted from the chair. This is a considerably easier task than directly lifting a limp, obese adolescent. Considerable psychologic and physiologic value is obtained from standing erect for at least several hours a day, aided by a tilt or standing table. Such activity reduces the frequency of static urinary complications and lessens the degree of osteoporosis.

Wheelchairs sometimes permit the home-confined walker the benefits of community travel. Electric wheelchairs are available for patients with insufficient strength to manage a standard model. These appliances require a van and lift for transport as they do not fold. Scoliosis pads or other external spinal containment measures are almost always necessary by the time a patient requires an electric apparatus. Centered hand controls are desirable, again to prevent leaning in the chair.

Upright mobility systems that combine the therapeutic benefits of vertical positioning with the locomotive advantages of a wheelchair (Fig 25–4) can sometimes be used in SMA, even when the patient lacks enough strength to move a wheelchair. In wheelchair-confined adult dystrophics, severe painful lordosis with marked increase in the lumbosacral angle sometimes occurs. This may require corseting for relief.

A portable electric, hydraulic, or mechanical lift facilitates care of

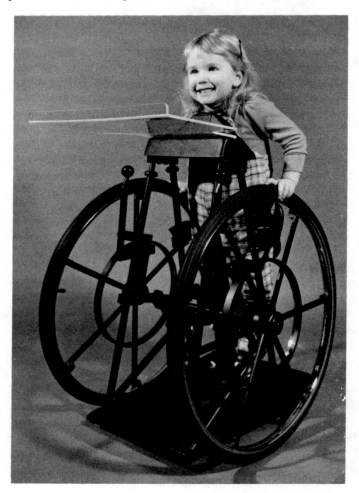

FIG 25–4.
Upright mobility system for SMA. (From Siegel I, Silverman M: Upright mobility system for spinal muscular atrophy patients. *Arch Phys Med Rehabil* 1984; 65:418. Used by permission.)

those patients who cannot transfer from chair to toilet or bed. Release of contractures with the application of braces may be desirable even though a patient is wheelchair confined. In long leg braces, the lower extremities can be locked in extension to avoid 90-degree knee flexion contractures. Another advantage of long leg braces is that they "set" the patient in his wheelchair, adding weight to the lower portion of the body, thus helping to maintain sitting balance by delaying pelvic tilt.

Complications frequently requiring management in wheelchair patients (Fig 25–5) include:

I. Scoliosis.
II. Obesity.
III. Acceleration of cardiopulmonary difficulties.
IV. Decrease in general rate of all metabolic processes.
V. Reduction of circulation to lower extremities with dependent edema.

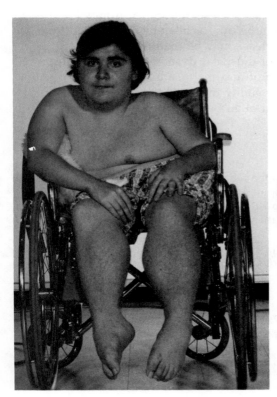

FIG 25–5.
Wheelchair-confined patients tend toward obesity, contractures, and scoliosis.

VI. Accelerating decrement of muscle mass, which reduces potassium stores. Sudden stress (such as infection) may result in sufficient loss of potassium to cause paralytic ileus.
VII. Increasing weakness and contracture.
    A. Normally, cardiac metabolism is greater in upper extremity work than in lower. Wheelchair locomotion requires 10% more energy expenditure than normal ambulation.
VIII. Sometimes mental and emotional problems secondary to confinement and almost complete lack of mobility.
IX. Functional problems of transfer, feeding and recreation, both for the patient and his family.
X. Possibility of superior mesenteric artery obstruction ("cast syndrome") secondary to constrictive torso bracing or (in thin individuals) when the patient with paralytic disease is moved to the sitting position.
XI. Increased incidence of vaginal infections due to difficulty with perineal toilet.
XII. Hip subluxation (or dislocation) seen in SMA groups I and II and advanced DMD can be uni- or bilateral and related to pelvic obliquity. Soft tissue release may be required for relief.

    Care at this stage of muscular dystrophy is truly "supportive." The preservation of maximal residual motor power and the maintenance of the ability to attend to TDL are important to both the patient's physical and emotional well-being.

BIBLIOGRAPHY

Abramson AS: An approach to the rehabilitation of children with muscular dystrophy. Muscular Dystrophy Association of America, Inc, Science Department, MDA Inc, Pub No 101, 1958.

Allen NR: Hearing acuity in patients with muscular dystrophy. *Dev Med Child Neurol* 1973; 15:500–505.

Chyatte SB, Long C, Vignos PJ, Jr: The balanced forearm orthosis in muscular dystrophy. *Arch Phys Med Rehabil* 1965; 46:633–636.

Gardner-Medwin D: Management of muscular dystrophy. *Physiotherapy* 1977; 63:46–51.

Gardner-Medwin D: Objectives in the management of Duchenne muscular dystrophy. *Isr J Med Sci* 1977; 13:229–234.

Garrett JM, DuBose TD, Jr, Jackson JE, et al: Esophageal and pulmonary disturbances in myotonia dystrophica. *Arch Intern Med* 1969; 123:26–32.

Hilliard Maj GD, Harris Co RE, Gilstrap Maj LC, et al: Myotonic muscular dystrophy in pregnancy. *South Med J* 1977; 70:446–452.

Huvos AG, Pruzanski W: Smooth muscle involvement in primary muscle disease. I. Myotonic dystrophy. *Arch Pathol* 1967; 83:229–233.

Huvos AG, Pruzanski W: Smooth muscle involvement in primary muscle disease. II. Progressive muscular dystrophy. *Arch Path* 1967; 83:234–240.

Ludman H: Dysphagia in dystrophia myotonica. *J Laryngol* 1962; 76:234–236.

Meyerson J, Lewis E, Ill K: Facioscapulohumeral muscular dystrophy and accompanying hearing loss. *Arch Otolaryngol* 1984; 110:261–266.

Mullendore JM, Stoudt RJ, Jr: Speech patterns of muscular dystrophic individuals. *J Speech Hear Disord* 1961; 26:252–257.

Robin GC, Falewski G: Acute gastric dilatation in progressive muscular dystrophy. *Lancet* 1963; 2:171–172.

Siegel IM: *The Clinical Management of Muscular Disease.* London, William Heinemann Medical Books Ltd, 1977.

26

Psychosocial

"Heredity sets limits; environment decides the exact position within these limits."

Edwin Carleton MacDowell (1887–1960)

"All happy families resemble one another; every unhappy family is unhappy in its own fashion."

Count Lyof Nikolayevitch Tolstoi (1828–1910), *Anna Karenina*, Part 1, Chapter 1

The importance of psychosocial care cannot be ignored in the treatment of neuromuscular disease because these conditions affect the psyche as well as the soma. Children with DMD face the same problems with peer interaction, body image, sexuality, and family adjustment that all normal children must resolve in the process of maturing. The major psychological tasks of adolescence are establishing emotional independence from parents, developing the capacity for lasting interpersonal relationships, and establishing a meaningful and stable identity, including a personal value system and commitment to a vocation. In order to accomplish this, the adolescent requires: an appropriate body image; new love objects; an available peer group; opportunity for learning; the ability to conceptualize (fantasize); and the willingness to try new roles.

The dystrophic adolescent is disabled by his disease, but "handicapped" by society. He is given few opportunities for independence. His nuclear (and extended) family may offer limited role models. He is forced to assume a dependent role. His normal sexual expression is thwarted. Caretakers often fail to distinguish between sexuality (feelings, drive, relationship processes) and sex acts (behavior). These problems are not unique, just exaggerated in the case of the disabled. The dystrophic child has increased difficulty establishing emotional independence from his parents. Because social contacts are limited, he frequently uses fantasy and denial as mechanisms of adjustment. Realistic but hopeful feedback (not pity) is required if the child is to develop a capacity for durable interpersonal relationships and an ability to establish the meaningful and stable identity that leads to self-acceptance. Sexual needs must be recognized and accepted, and the home should provide appropriate role models, privacy, and opportunity for learning.

Psychiatric intervention that is supportive and made available at times of psychologic crisis can avert critical emotional damage. Such times are (1) when the diagnosis is first made, (2) when the child realizes he is different from other children because of increasing difficulty with motor tasks (usually about age 7), (3) when bracing becomes necessary, and (4) when the child becomes wheelchair confined. Empathetic and intelligent counseling of both the patient and the family throughout the course of the illness is an important part of the total management of the disease. This includes early discovery of carriers and appropriate genetic counseling of both the parents and female siblings. Guilt is often felt by and projected to the female because of the X-linked nature of the genetic transmission. Responsibility, of course, should be shared between both father and mother if for no other reason than the fact that the father determines the sex of the child.

Factors in the psychosocial management of the patient and his family include the following:

I. Realistic expectations.
   A. The specific limitations imposed by the disease must be recognized and a life space provided for patients so they may live productively and as normally as possible. Honest expectations should be set for these children, as is the case with any crippling disease.
   B. Overprotection must be avoided, allowing the child to accomplish by his own efforts those tasks that win the approbation of his environment.
      1. Such overprotection, rather than helping, inevitably leads to isolation and dependency.

    2. Thus, such children should be "mainstreamed" as long as feasible.

    3. Where appropriate, vocational training should be geared toward a career enabling the child to undertake an occupation within the limits of his disability.

C. There are no distinct psychopathologic entities exclusive to muscular dystrophy, and severe emotional illness is no more common than in a normal population.

    1. Because progressive disability is so devastatingly overwhelming, any psychological defense mechanism that is not harmful should not be discouraged.

D. The association of muscular dystrophy and lowered intelligence quotient has been documented.

    1. Intellectual retardation has been observed in 30% to 50% of patients with DMD (Fig 26–1).

      a) Verbal scores are affected more than performance functioning.

      b) The intellectual subnormality is present from birth and is nonprogressive. It appears unrelated to whether or not the disease is hereditary or spontaneous.

      c) In a family containing two or more patients, the affected members often have a similar IQ, suggesting that mental retardation may be genetically determined.

      d) A greater than normal incidence of diffuse EEG abnormalities has been reported in DMD.

      e) Although retardation may be related to an organic etiology in DMD, lowered IQ may also reflect depressed functioning secondary to the psychological, social, and educational impositions of the disease that prevent pa-

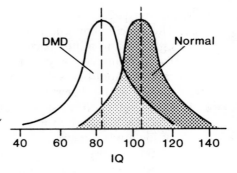

FIG 26–1.
Distribution curves of IQ in DMD and normal subjects. (Modified from Dubowitz V: *Mental Retardation in Duchenne Muscular Dystrophy.* Amsterdam, Excerpta Medica, International Congress Series No. 404, 1977.)

tients from realizing their intellectual potential. Learning disabilities are frequent.

 f) Decreased intellectual functioning does not occur in patients with limb-girdle or FSH dystrophy. Mental defects, hypersomnia, sociopathic behavior, intellectual deterioration, and lack of initiative are often present in varying degrees in dystrophia myotonica. A "belle indifference" as well as mild paranoia have been noted. Nonspecific EEG abnormalities, cerebral ventricular enlargement, and cerebral heterotopias have also been described in this disease.

 E. Patients with DMD typically:
  1. Are emotionally dependent and lack frustration tolerance.
  2. Tend toward social and emotional withdrawal and, failing to develop dominant modes of conscious attitudes, favor emotional seesawing and impulsive responses.

 F. The family dealing with a handicapped child need not necessarily become a handicapped family. Due to the psychological aspects of chronic illness, disease in a child represents a family crisis. How this crisis is resolved depends in great part on the preexisting strength of the family unit. It requires considerable vigor, stability, resilience, and powers of adjustment to sustain a muscular dystrophic child in a family. Assessment of the existence and use of professional support systems is a vital function of family-centered care.

II. Factors in the management of a dystrophic child and his family include:
 A. The child's personality as well as his needs.
 B. The child's stage of emotional development and his vulnerabilities.
 C. The child's perception of his illness and its management.
 D. The nature of the disease itself and its potential effects on the patient and his family.
 E. The nature of the management procedure and the potential for support of the child from his family and physician.

III. The adjustment of a young patient with muscular dystrophy can be affected by several factors, including:
 A. The requirement for parental separation at any time during the disease. Young children separated for long periods of time from parents show adverse reactions, characterized by a stage of protest, followed by a stage of detachment or denial.
 B. Restriction, including sensory impairment and isolation.

When the normal avenues for expression through play are restricted, a child may withdraw into excessive fantasy as a means of coping.
  C. Lack of consistency and dependency.
  D. Deformity and pain. This includes the threat of surgery and concerns over being defective, hence the fear of becoming an inadequate person.
  E. The threat of death. It is not usually until age 9 or 10 that a child fully understands death as being both inevitable and irrevocable.
  F. Medication. Prolonged, regular use of drugs may be regarded as an imposition by authority figures.
  G. Absence from school.
IV. The following factors influence the family's response to the severe stress on the family unit of coping with the diagnosis and treatment of a chronic, crippling illness in one of its members:
  A. The severity of the illness, including both the prognosis and the availability of an effective treatment.
  B. Whether or not the disease is congenital.
  C. The age of onset of the disease and the age at which the diagnosis is made.
  D. The presence of a preexisting emotional disturbance within the family.
  E. The nature and effects of the illness itself.
  F. The effects of a program of home management and restrictions on family life.
  G. The presence or absence of affected siblings.
  H. The stress of repeated hospitalizations and surgical procedures.
  I. The cost of the illness, if privately treated.

Specific emotional responses seen in parents include denial, anxiety, feelings of guilt, depression, resentment (and rejection), and reactions of shame, embarrassment, or sheer exhaustion.

Many parent pairs evolve through the various stages of mourning after learning the diagnosis. This includes a period of disbelief and denial, succeeded by one of anger and rage, followed by bargaining and, finally, acceptance and adjustment. Because (in DMD particularly) there are a number of critical psychosocial incidents (as mentioned before, diagnosis, inability of the patient to cope, bracing, wheelchair confinement, etc.), parents may reinitiate the mourning process at each of these stages.

Sibling reactions are more or less characterized by similar emotional states. Normal siblings often feel either responsible for their diseased siblings and/or guilty over their own normality. Concerning muscular dystrophy, the disease may largely form the basis for a family's way of life; due to the demands of the illness, siblings become "handicapped" in the struggle for parental affection and attention. A sibship is unique in that it can span six or more decades. Siblings identify closely with each other. They may feel responsible for each other's well-being. The healthy child must be aided in developing his own identity and in understanding the differences and similarities between himself and his disabled sibling. Systematic and routine inquiry should be made into the effect the illness may be having on normal siblings. Specific information regarding peer relationships, academic progress, sleep, mood, etc. should be sought. These feelings are difficult to approach with ordinary interviewing techniques. Projective testing (such as the kinetic family drawing test—K-F-D) has been used as a diagnostic procedure for evaluating interpersonal dynamics in families with muscular dystrophy. Through such testing, attitudes and conflicts of both children with dystrophy and their normal siblings are evoked and compared. Unaffected siblings demonstrate anger and depression in ways that would not have easily been identified in clinical interviews alone. Use of projective testing can aid in programming treatment for these families.

What the family needs is empathy, not sympathy, detachment rather than avoidance. Whatever the physician's reaction, he should realize this.

V. The management of the family with a muscular dystrophic child or children is based on a recognition that such a situation will have major implications on the life of that family. Diagnosis can easily precipitate a state of familial crisis. The family's history of adjustment may give clues to the nature of potential difficulties. The health professional dealing with such a family must recognize that what they hear and understand may differ considerably from what they have been told. In general, the family can understand only what they are prepared for emotionally. One must maintain regular visits with the family in order to clarify what they have heard regarding diagnosis, prognosis, and management, and to supervise their day-to-day coping with management problems, both physical and emotional. At the same time, the expression of anxiety on the part of both the dystrophic child and his normal siblings must be facilitated.

Group therapy has proved valuable in assisting parents of children with neuromuscular disease by helping them develop insight and increasing communication through sharing of experiences. Through such groups, parents learn to recognize their own attitudes and acknowledge that the focus of their attention is on a process they can't stop. They begin to accept the situation more realistically and to concentrate on areas of their lives they can influence. In general, parents of children with muscular dystrophy have low expectations of their ability to cope, and they defend themselves against testing these abilities. They isolate themselves from reminders of the future and ignore the developmental and emotional problems of their child, such as difficulties with independence or sexuality. Rather, they focus on the physical problems of the disease. Once they recognize that the anticipation of progressive limitation is the greatest fear, they can learn to accept themselves and their children and to respond to problem situations more honestly.

Parents with less disabled children are more anxious about future limitations, but are also aware of the developmental problems their children currently face. Parents with more severely disabled children seem to be less anxious about the future but also appear to have suppressed consciousness of the developmental problems their children continue to encounter. All parents obstruct their awareness by concentrating on the physical aspects and limitations brought on by the disease.

Although psychosocial problems faced by parents of children with neuromuscular disease are somewhat similar, their timing is different. Parents of children with DMD are able to prolong denial of their child's premature death because the child's loss of function is gradual. In contrast, parents of children with SMA go through an initial phase of mourning that eventually enables them to be open to a wider range of life experiences as they become accustomed to their child's survival. Parents of SMA children encounter similar difficulties regardless of the age of their children. A child with SMA at age 3 is much like a child with SMA at age 10. It is likely that both may be confined to a wheelchair. In contrast, a dystrophic child at age 3 appears to be almost normal, whereas by age 10 such a child may well be in a wheelchair. Also, SMA children differ from DMD children in several ways that influence the responses of their parents: (1) SMA children are usually of normal or above normal intelligence; (2) mental retardation has been reported in a significant number of children with DMD; and (3) children confined to wheelchairs appear to be more observant of their immediate surroundings than children who are ambulatory.

Parents of dystrophic children seem to have more difficulty in dealing with the psychosocial problems of their child, whereas parents of SMA children have more difficulty delineating parenting roles. Parents of SMA children more readily accept equal responsibility for the birth of their handicapped child (this being an autosomal recessive disease). Both groups of parents are strongly influenced by relatives and doctors. Relatives and friends have the greatest influence in helping define parenting skills.

Health professionals should make their interventions appropriate to the different stages of these and other diseases with similar characteristics. A liaison should also be maintained with the child's school, as peer relationships are extremely important in his day to day life.

Physicians must realize that they are frequently the objects of a hostility that is not personally directed. Rather, it is a displacement of both the patient's and the parents' resentment toward the fact of the child's illness and a reaction against the one who is confronting them with painful realities they would rather not face. Physicians who respond with hostility or withdrawal to these projected feelings will lose the valuable opportunity of providing needed services at a time of great stress. Doctors should be aware of the syndrome of professional (as well as parental) burnout in the management of these difficult problems.

VI. Parents of dystrophic children are faced with serious problems of adjustment. Feelings of guilt, leading to penance and a life of servitude to the child, may contribute to the vicious cycle of guilt, anger, self-pity, and ultimate rejection, both of self and the patient. In the X-linked form of the disease, such feelings are more prevalent in the mother. Fathers, on the other hand, because of their work routines, are less disrupted by the presence of a seriously ill, homebound child, and because they may feel less responsible in the production of a sex-linked mutation, seem to bear less primary guilt, but frequently more anger and self-pity.

Demands on the mother's time and strength are severe. Neighbors are not always tactful, and strangers provoke self-consciousness and shame. Normal siblings are often neglected and indeed, part of a counselor's job is to help parents realize the prospects of the dystrophic child in his home situation as well as his limitations, and to aid siblings who have to compete with a sick child for parental attention. Early discovery of carriers and appropriate genetic counseling are necessary to allay anxiety over the hereditary implications of these diseases that disturb parents and siblings alike.

The nature of Duchenne muscular dystrophy demands a unique pattern of adjustment, and a careful understanding of it is essential for providing clinical care.

A. Parents of children with DMD are significantly concerned with problems relating to the care of their dystrophic child, often at the expense of other personal relationships and to the exclusion of other family needs.

B. For mothers in particular, it appears that the more the problems of the disease are openly acknowledged, the harder it is to cope. Frequent participation in activities with the child, rather than facilitating adaptation by alleviating isolation, contributes to the pressure felt. Expeditious changes that must be made, even if they ease situational problems, have the overall effect of increasing the difficulties of coping.

C. Fathers are less involved with the ongoing care of the dystrophic child; consequently, coping is less clearly related to the same factors for them as for mothers. On the other hand, problems for fathers are more frequently stage-specific. Mothers are more involved early, and it becomes harder for them sooner. For fathers, the difficulties are more keenly felt later.

D. The value of marital stability for both husbands and wives cannot be overemphasized. If for no other reason, the sheer complexity of dealing with the physical work involved in caring for a dystrophic child (particularly as he becomes older and the disease progresses) contributes to the importance of remaining married.

E. Enormous concern for the physical work necessary to care for the dystrophic child is present. The expressed need and desire for help in child care is substantial.

F. Therapeutic implications of the above are clear:

   1. Parents should be allowed to focus some of their attention and energy on each other and on the unaffected children in the family.

   2. Intervention should be aimed at increased, earlier involvement of fathers in the care of the child.

    3. One must understand the importance of marital stability and concentrate on other aspects of the marital relationship.

    4. The amount of physical work demanded of the parents (the mother in particular) should be alleviated. Child care services must be available.

    5. *Progressive* integration and *gradual* acceptance facilitate adaptation. As noted, parents of children with DMD often go through a new sequence of coping with each stage of the disease. One level of disability is accepted, assimilated, and internalized just as a transition to the next occurs. Thus, understanding and allowing *prolonged* reworking of the coping tasks is an important implication for clinical care.

VII. The treating physician must offer intelligent and empathetic advice, correlating definitive therapy with an ongoing program of understanding and patient and parent counseling during the early (diagnostic) phase of treatment. Information should be available to parents on demand. Often, patients, parents, and professionals do not perceive the same issues as being important. Particular care must be taken to see that no credibility gap occurs and there is no delay in diagnosis. Pastoral counseling is often helpful in providing spiritual support and dealing with existential concerns such as, "why me?," death, etc. Many parents, shocked by a diagnosis of DMD, will panic and spend useless energy, time, and funds seeking a diagnosis with a better prognosis. The physician making the initial diagnosis should discuss "shopping" with all parents. They should be encouraged to get a reputable second opinion, but also advised to return to the primary physician. The hereditary implications of the disease can be briefly discussed during an early interview. Available treatment should be outlined and parents encouraged that research is being conducted in the search for the cause and cure of the disease. One must be prepared emotionally and have enough time to listen to anxious parents unburden themselves. During long-term follow-up, such matters as the following can be discussed:

    A. Sibling responsibility and responsibility to siblings.

    B. Methods of coping in the home.

    C. Instruction in how to listen well, how to "tune in" to a child's problems, and how to "read between the lines."

    D. Discussion of the dystrophic child's most common worries, including concern over the trouble he might be causing. Judicious use of motorized lifts and other aids for daily living may go far in alleviating such concern.

E. Instruction in the usual psychosocial dynamics of the situation (e.g., guilt causing overprotectiveness).

F. Teaching parents to use their intuition. Parents should be told that even though they have no ready solution, just indicating that they recognize the problem can go a long way toward solving it.

When patients inquire about the disease, including its fatal aspect, they must be given answers commensurate with their understanding that are realistic yet hopeful. It is important to recognize exactly what the child is asking and respond to this specific request for information, and not to one's own anxieties and fantasies.

At the point that a muscular dystrophic can no longer attend school and becomes home-bound, parents must face the ultimate painful recognition of the severity of the child's condition. Also, the mother is now occupied with the patient all day long. The father will often feel guilt in relation to the mother, who is so heavily beset by the everyday physical and psychological problems of the child. This guilt stems from the fact that the father is less involved in this drudgery and, secretly and understandably, relieved that it is not he who is bearing the brunt of the problem. Empathic intervention at this point can often deter a severe parental crisis.

During the early course of the disease, the patient should be asked what he has been told by his teachers, siblings, parents, and peers; a frank discussion of his concerns should be initiated. A simple explanation of muscular dystrophy can be given. One must be truthful but optimistic. The patient has to be encouraged to unburden himself of fears and fantasies, and the doctor must be a good listener.

Illness in adolescence is resented as a particularly painful cheating of someone about to experience all the supposed freedoms and opportunities that attend adult status. Informative pamphlets and other literature provided by the Muscular Dystrophy Association are helpful in both patient and family education. Peer support groups organized by local MDA chapters have proven of significant assistance to many parents in coping with the physical and psychosocial problems of the disease. Professional counseling of individuals and families has been of inestimable value.

As mentioned, it is desirable to keep the child in a regular school as long as possible. It is best if the school is close to home, so the child can be with his friends. Vacation and after-school activities are thereby enhanced. This arrangement requires the understanding and cooperation of the principal and teachers. A telephone call from the physician can often clarify matters and gain this cooperation.

Preventive psychiatry can be employed, particularly during puberty. At this time, fantasies run rampant and should be discussed. Aggression and denial are also apparent in this phase and require attention. One must discuss feelings of dependency on the mother, the need for privacy, and the matter of masturbation. Adolescents often display significant isolation and difficulty discussing issues such as death with their parents. At the same time, parents find it difficult to respond to death issues with their dystrophic sons—a reaction that leaves the boys alone and the parents guilty.

Where a physician feels unprepared or unable to handle these matters, both parents and child should be referred to an appropriate person (psychologist, social worker, psychiatrist) or agency where such help is available.

Attention paid to the psychosocial aspects of muscular dystrophy can add productive life to the years available to these patients. In the treatment of muscular dystrophy, the family is indeed the patient.

BIBLIOGRAPHY

Anderson F, Bardach J, Goodgold J: Sexuality and neuromuscular disease. (Rehab Mono #56). Institute of Rehabilitative Medicine and Muscular Dystrophy Association, New York, 1979.

Black FW: Intellectual ability as related to age and stage of disease in muscular dystrophy: A brief note. *J Psychol* 1973; 84:333–334.

Botvin-Madorsky JG, Radford LM, Neumann EM: Psychosocial aspects of death and dying in Duchenne muscular dystrophy. *Arch Phys Med Rehabil* 1984; 65:79–82.

Bowlby J: *Separation Anxiety and Anger: Attachment and Loss*, vol 2. New York, Basic Books, 1973, pp 3–24.

Bregman AM: Living with progressive childhood illness: parental management of neuromuscular disease. *Soc Work Health Care* 1980; 5:387–407.

Buchanan DC, LaBarbera CJ, Roelofs R, et al: Reactions of families to children with Duchenne muscular dystrophy. *Gen Hosp Psychiatry* 1979; 1:263–269.

Cain AC, Fast I, Erickson ME: Children's disturbed reactions to the death of a sibling. *Am J Orthopsychiatry* 1964; 34:741–752.

Dubowitz V: Intellectual impairment in muscular dystrophy. *Arch Dis Child* 1965; 40:296–301.

Firth M, Gardner-Medwin D, Hosking G, et al: Interviews with parents of boys suffering from Duchenne muscular dystrophy. *Dev Med Child Neurol* 1983; 25:466–471.

Freedman AM, Helme W, Havel J, et al: Psychiatric aspects of familial dysautonomia. *Am J Orthopsychiatry* 1957; 27:96–106.

Holroyd J, Guthrie D: Stress in families of children with neuromuscular disease. *J Clin Psych* 1979; 35:734–739.

Kornfeld M, Siegel IM: Parental group therapy in the management of a fatal childhood disease. *Health Soc Work* 1979; 4:99–118.

Leibowitz D, Dubowitz V: Intellect and behavior in Duchenne muscular dystrophy. *Dev Med Child Neurol* 1981; 23:577–590.

Marsh GG, Munsat TL: Evidence for early impairment of verbal intelligence in Duchenne muscular dystrophy. *Arch Dis Child* 1974; 49:118–122.

Rossman NP, Kakulas BA: Mental deficiency associated with muscular dystrophy: A neuropathological study. *Brain* 1966; 89:769–787.

Siegel IM, Davidson H, Kornfeld M, et al: Coping with muscular dystrophy: Psychosocial correlates of adaptation. *Muscle Nerve* 1983; 6:607–609.

Siegel IM, Kornfeld MS: Some aspects of parental group therapy in the management of spinal muscular atrophy, in Gamstrop I, Sarnat H (eds): *Progressive Spinal Muscular Atrophies*. New York, Raven Press, 1984, pp 189–199.

Siegel IM, Kornfeld MS: Kinetic family drawing test for evaluating families having children with muscular dystrophy. *J Am Phys Ther* 1980; 60:293–298.

Steinhauer PD, Mushin DN, Rae-Grant Q: Psychological aspects of chronic illness. *Pediatr Clin North Am* 1974; 21:825–840.

Taft LT: The care and management of the child with muscular dystrophy. *Dev Med Child Neurol* 1973; 15:510–518.

Tomonaga M, Muro T, Kito S: Intelligence scale and electroencephalographic findings on the progressive muscular dystrophy. *Iryo* 1967; 21:800–806.

Witte RA: The psychosocial impact of a progressive physical handicap and terminal illness (Duchenne muscular dystrophy) on adolescents and their families. *Br J Med Psych* 1985; 58:179–187.

Worden DK, Vignos PJ, Jr: Intellectual functions in childhood progressive muscular dystrophy. *Pediatrics* 1962; 29:968–977.

27

Summary

"Things should be made as simple as possible, but no simpler."
Albert Einstein (1879–1955)

Muscle is under CNS control. It is profoundly influenced by peripheral nerve function. Excitation occurs through its membrane system and contraction by way of ionic changes mediated within the SR-T tubular complex to the coupling of actin and myosin modulated by the troponin-tropomyosin diad. Its metabolism is either glycolytic or oxidative. Necessary fuel is processed by the muscle mitochondria and spent through the ATP-ADP sequence.

SYSTEMS ANALYSIS OF MUSCLE

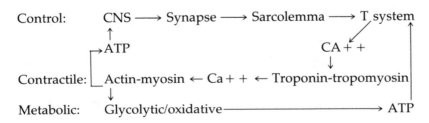

Control: CNS ⟶ Synapse ⟶ Sarcolemma ⟶ T system

Contractile: Actin-myosin ← Ca + + ← Troponin-tropomyosin

Metabolic: Glycolytic/oxidative ⟶ ATP

1. Muscular dystrophy is the general designation for a group of chronic diseases whose most prominent characteristic is a progressive degeneration of skeletal musculature.

2. Although any of the voluntary muscles can be affected, axial musculature and that of the limb girdles is most frequently and most profoundly involved.

3. Diseases of skeletal muscle are for the most part hereditary conditions, though spontaneous occurrence as a result of genetic neomutation is common.

4. As a general rule, the earlier clinical symptoms appear, the more rapid is the progression of the disease.

5. The primary pathology in all types of dystrophy appears to lie in the muscle cell itself. However, the nervous system may be indirectly involved.

6. No treatment has been found to correct the underlying pathology, nor to arrest the relentless progression in the majority of muscular dystrophies.

7. A knowledge of these diseases, their differential diagnosis, and their ergonomics and dynamics is important for purposes of treatment, prognosis, detection of carriers in the X-linked varieties, and genetic counseling.

8. Diagnosis need not entirely depend on history and clinical examination alone. Electrodiagnosis is available, as well as serum muscle enzyme quantification and muscle biopsy.

9. Management should be prospective, consisting of supportive and symptomatic therapy with particular attention paid to cardiomyopathy, pulmonary complications, nutritional needs, functional treatment of fractures, and psychological and social problems. A means of referral, information, coordination of services, advocacy, and continued family support should be provided.

10. The patient and his family should be educated in the legal rights of the disabled to employment, health care, and social and rehabilitation services provided by local, state, and federal services.

11. Serial assessment helps in determining the functional stage of the disease and indicating specific therapies.

12. Occupational therapy, by applying optimization techniques to maximize performance, is utilized to assist the patient in meeting the

needs of his activities of daily living within the restrictions imposed by his disease.

13. Physical therapy aids in augmenting and utilizing residual strength and relieving contractures through passive stretch.

14. Through an understanding of the postural pathomechanics, kinematics, and energetics of these diseases, orthopedics provides procedures for the surgical release of lower extremity contractures, the repair of foot and ankle deformity, in selected cases the operative treatment of scoliosis, stabilization of the shoulders, and other rational methods for avoiding or correcting skeletal distortion.

15. Progressive disability can be delayed by a variety of physiatric techniques, including the prescription of appropriate orthoses.

16. When no longer ambulatory, patients require wheelchairs and a variety of special devices to facilitate ongoing care.

17. Proper treatment of the patient with muscle disease is multidisciplined and aggressive. Although the disease disables the patient, it is often society that handicaps him. Continued education and agitation for acceptance and equal opportunity (architectural access, employment, etc.) are important facets of holistic therapy.

18. Through a program of thoughtful care, the frustrating aspects of these conditions can be minimized while maximizing the benefits obtained through available therapies, increasing comfort and function and enabling the patient to live as fully as possible for as long as feasible.

Index